Social Workers
in Health Care Management:
The Move to Leadership

Contributors

Susan S. Bailis, MSW, Executive Vice President, ADS Management, Inc., Lawrence, MA 01845

Sylvia S. Clarke, MSc, Consultant, Department of Social Work Services, The Mount Sinai Hospital, New York, NY 10029, and Editor, *Social Work in Health Care*

Marybeth Flower, LCSW, Administrator, Division of Education, Pacific Presbyterian Medical Center, San Francisco, CA 94120

Steven J. Goe, MSW, Administrator, Scripps Memorial Hospital, Encinitas, CA 92020

Karil S. Klingbeil, MSW, Assistant Professor, School of Social Work, Assistant Administrator and Director of Social Work, Harborview Medical Center, University of Washington, Seattle, WA 98104

Harold L. Light, MSS, President, The Long Island College Hospital, Brooklyn, NY 11201

Stanley K. Nielsen, ACSW, Director, Patient and Family Services, Meritor/Madison General Hospital, 202 South Park Street, Madison, WI 53715

Gary Rosenberg, PhD, Edith J. Baerwald Professor of Community Medicine (Social Work), Mt. Sinai School of Medicine; Director, Department of Social Work Services, Mt. Sinai Hospital; Vice President of Human Resources, Mt. Sinai Medical Center, New York, NY 10029

W. June Simmons, LCSW, Director, Senior Care Network, Huntington Memorial Hospital, Pasadena, CA 91105

Patricia J. Volland, MSW, MBA, Vice President, Planning and Development, Deaton Hospital and Medical Center, Baltimore, MD 21230

Saul Zeichner, MSW, ACSW, Vice President, Administration, Mt. Kemble Division, Morristown Memorial Hospital, Morristown, NJ 07960

Social Workers in Health Care Management: The Move to Leadership

Gary Rosenberg, PhD
Sylvia S. Clarke, MSc
Editors

The Haworth Press
New York • London

Social Workers in Health Care Management: The Move to Leadership has also been published as *Social Work in Health Care*, Volume 12, Number 3, Spring 1987.

Library of Congress Cataloging-in-Publication Data

Social workers in health care management.

Also published as: Social work in health care; v. 12, no. 3 (spring 1987)
Includes bibliographies.
1. Medical social work—United States—Administration. 2. Hospitals—United States—Adminis-
tration. I. Rosenberg, Gary. II. Clarke, Sylvia S. [DNLM: 1. Community Health Services—organi-
zation & administration. 2. Delivery of Health Care—organization & administration. 3. Hospital
Administration. 4. Leadership. 5. Social Work—organization & administration. W1 S0135P v.12
no.3 / W 322 S6765]
HV687.5.U5S654   1988   362.1'1'068   87-15026
ISBN 0-86656-672-4
ISBN 0-86656-815-8 (pbk.)

Social Workers in Health Care Management: The Move to Leadership

CONTENTS

CHAPTER XII

Findings and Implications   **143**
Gary Rosenberg, PhD
Sylvia S. Clarke, MSc

Somehow, working in a field other than traditional social work is viewed as having "left the profession." It is also a fact that few who "leave" continue to identify with the profession whose skills they employ.

On the other hand, it is possible that until now the utility of social work education—in contrast to law, accounting, and others—has been so narrowly focused as to limit employment opportunity in other fields. Perhaps consideration should be given to loosening the stricture to allow a place for alternate careers that involve such social work skills as interviewing, conflict resolution, group dynamics, and others. Making this possible will require both a clearer definition of social work knowledge and skills and an identification of the opportunities for their broader application.

Samuel J. Silberman
"A View From the Sidelines"
Council on Social Work Education
Thirtieth Annual Meeting
Second Plenary Session
March 12, 1984

CHAPTER I

The Study:
Purpose and Method

Over the past decade a significant number of hospital social work
anagers have moved to broader management responsibilities in health
re settings. The impetus for this study is the wish to understand this
enomenon. What are the positives and problems in this "upward"
ovement? Are there conflicts? What is their nature? What are the
dvantages? Are social work's values subject to compromise, to ethical
lemmas? What transitional stresses are involved in moving from the
anagement of a resource service area to executive level management?

As the senior editor himself moved in this direction and took
sponsibility for managing several other hospital functions in addition to
s job of directing the social work department, many colleagues raised
ese issues and posed dilemmas they saw or feared.

Some of them were seeking or had been offered similar opportunities.
ere they "selling out" social work, "leaving it behind" to "move
ead"? Were they abandoning their profession? How did their col-
agues view their professionalism? Should and could they maintain
sponsibility for the social work operation and at the same time direct
nd manage other areas? Are such dual responsibilities basically conflict-
g or can they be congruent? Is one's professional identity lost, diluted
r enhanced?

As opportunities in hospital management increased and these questions
roliferated, we came to think that a careful examination of these issues
as indicated. The body of experiences already accrued by these
xecutive hospital colleagues could provide a base for new knowledge.
his volume is an exploratory study of these experiences. We did not
xpect this exploratory study would provide conclusive answers to the

1

questions raised and have tried in our concluding chapter to distil issu
and questions for further study and research.

To give direction to the study, we reviewed the work of Levinson ar
Clurman (1972), Rino Patti (1983, 1979, 1977), Patti and Rauch (1978
Patti and Austin (1977) who have studied the transitions of clinicians
managers. This led us to the major goals of this study:

— to examine the experiences of a small group of social wor
    directors now carrying hospital executive functions;
— to identify their commonalities and differences;
— to pinpoint themes, issues and dilemmas as precisely as possibl
    and
— to identify areas for further study.

We were interested, too, in seeing whether and how social wor
education is helpful in the transition from social work to hospit;
manager. Questions have been raised for some time about whether shift
are needed in the curricula of graduate school of social work to bette
prepare and support all social work practitioners for possible future caree
moves into management positions in any social agency. This is
universal career track for many social workers. Is it functional for th
MSW curriculum to prepare individuals to manage non-social wor
functions?

In the selection of a sample, we invited 14 out of an unknow
population of outstanding social workers who were executive managers i
hospital settings to participate in the project with us. We do not know i
the sample is representative or quantitatively reliable. We assume tha
there are a number of other colleagues who could have participated too
they were not included simply because we did not know them. We
reached out to participants primarily through personal contacts as well a;
through our connections with the Society for Hospital Social Work
Directors of the American Hospital Association, an organization that ha;
provided a productive forum for stimulating social work leaders in the
development of their management skills.

Eleven of the 14 agreed to join us in the project; and the work of 10
comprise the basic data we examined and the bulk of the book. The
eleventh, Eleanor Clark, of the Massachusetts General Hospital, who had
encouraged us to undertake this work, could not make her contribution
because of her untimely death. We miss her and her wisdom.

We developed an outline for the contributors to use as a guide to their
narratives. We wanted them to cover content areas which were as uniform
as possible but we did not want to restrict their conceptual or writing
styles. We listed the areas we thought needed to be addressed for study

rposes and left them free to deal with them as they wished, to add or
btract, expand or contract as was relevant to their experiences.

We asked for a description of their current positions and scope of their
sponsibilities. We wanted to learn whether they continued as manager
the social work department; if not, whether it is one of the programs
r which they are accountable; or whether they are institutional managers
ith no official tie to the social work department.

We suggested that they tell us how they came to assume these new
sponsibilities. Did they move out and plan for the move? Did the
stitution reach out to them? Why? What were their motivations in
oving to this new arena?

Other queries were directed to what aspects of social work knowledge,
ills and values they found germane and useful in the responsibilities
ey now carry. How and in what ways does being a social worker help
em be an able manager? In what ways, if any, is it impedimental? What
ills that they already possessed were useful and easily transferred to
eir new positions? What additional knowledge and skills did they need
acquire? Were additional formal credentials needed? What did they
xperience as positives in their moves? What difficulties and problems
id they encounter?

We asked them if they could draw conclusions from their experiences.
Vhat do they think are implications for social work practice, education
nd research?

The reader will see how, despite the uniform outline, each contributor
eveloped a unique and vivid document. We are indebted to them for
eir willingness to share their experiences and to develop conceptualiza-
ons of their practice in written form.

Their ten chapters follow alphabetically, by author. In the last chapter
e editors have tried to synthesize what these essays have taught us and
ote what we need to study further.

Gary Rosenberg, PhD
Sylvia S. Clarke, MSc

REFERENCES

evinson, Daniel J. and Clurman, Gerald L. "The Clinician Executive," *Administration in Mental Health*, Winter, 1972, pp. 53–67.

atti, Rino J. "Social Welfare Administration," *Managing Social Programs in a Developmental Context*, Englewood Cliffs, N.J.: Prentice-Hall, 1983.

atti, Rino J. "Patterns of Management Activity in Social Welfare Agencies," *Administration in Social Work*, Vol. 1, No. 1, Spring 1977, pp. 5–18.

atti, Rino J. et al., "From Direct Service to Administration: A Study of Social Workers Transitions from Clinical to Management Roles," *Administration in Social Work*, Vol. 3, No. 2, Summer 1979, pp. 131–151.

Patti, Rino J. et al., "From Direct Service to Administration: A Study of Social Workers Transitic from Clinical to Management Roles, Part II, Recommendations," *Administration in Social Wo* Vol. 3, No. 3, Fall 1979, pp. 165–275.

Patti, Rino J., and Rausch, Robert. "Social Work Administration: Graduates in the Job Market, *F* Analysis of Managers Hiring Preferences," *Social Service Review*, December 1978, p 567–583.

Patti, Rino J., and Austin, Michael J. "Socializing the Direct Service Practitioner in the Ways Supervisory Management," *Administration in Social Work*, Vol. 1, No. 3, Fall 1977, p 267–280.

CHAPTER II

Reflections on a Journey

Susan S. Bailis, MSW, ACSW

My comments about social workers as administrators in health care settings are less a theoretical examination of the applicability of social work skills to health care administration or a "how to" for advancement in the hospital, but rather more of a personal review of career evolution. This evolution occurred for me, partly as the result of the changing options for women, partly from my liberation of ambitions and wishes, and partly from the availability of opportunities at the right place and time.

CURRENT RESPONSIBILITIES

I am the Associate Director of New England Medical Center as well as the Director of Social Work Services.* This places me in the senior management of an academic medical center with a wide scope of responsibilities besides social work. My administrative responsibilities include the emergency room, a walk-in clinic, a nutrition center, a contract with a neighborhood health center, quality assurance, infection control, an employee assistance program, interpreter service, the patient representative function and a leadership role in new ventures and acquisitions. I manage approximately 100 people and a four million dollar budget. In addition to my "line" responsibilities, I hold "staff" responsibilities in the hospital as well, as a participant in a variety of efforts such as vertical integration and other long-range planning concerns, medical staff organizational issues, and outside regulatory response.

*Ms. Bailis is now Executive Vice President of ADS Management, Inc. Lawrence, MA.

With this litany of responsibilities, one might justifiably question why I have held on to the social work directorship. This is a question that helps to illuminate the key issues faced by many social workers who look at career evolution in health care settings. There are advantages and disadvantages to retaining the leadership of the social work function and a good case can be made for making either decision—if one is given the choice. Not all social work directors who move into administrative positions have that latitude. I have had flexibility with that decision, although my institution's lack of initiative in urging me to relinquish the directorship may well have frugality at its roots rather than management theory. If I explore why I have elected to maintain my role as the director of social work service, despite the fact that only 20%–30% of my time now goes to the social work department, the answer lies as much in identity as anything. To give up being director of social work service hints at relinquishing my social work identity in the hospital.

DUAL RESPONSIBILITIES—A PERSONAL PERSPECTIVE

I believe strongly that the *potential* role of social work is much broader than the traditional one of clinical social work practice in a department. Despite this belief, I have a nagging worry about giving up the directorship of the department as I feel I will be relinquishing a piece of my identity as a social worker. Thus my argument in regard to identity is not so much rational as it is emotional.

However, there are some rational factors related to maintaining the directorship role. Social work directors can exercise greater control and involvement over the social work function than their nominal superiors, thereby directly having an impact on programs in a way that cannot happen in purely an administrative position. The distance that comes with high level administration is a loss that is not necessarily a price that needs to be paid.

Another reason for retaining the social work directorship is that holding a high level administrative position in a hospital is a much higher risk situation. When the chief executive officer leaves, his or her successor may want a new senior management team. Being a director of social work is not dissimilar from tenure in a university. A high level administrative position in no way comes with tenure, but rather tends to rise and fall based on relationships with top management. I have no illusions that my power in the hospital is directly related to the reality of my relationships with top management. Should top management change, so might my position. Yet I do not think that I fully protect myself by holding dual titles. I would not want to go back to spending all of my time as director of social work at this point in my career.

DUAL RESPONSIBILITIES—THE SOCIAL WORK DEVELOPMENT PERSPECTIVE

I think the social work department benefits and suffers from my dual responsibilities. It gets the benefit of additional power, access, and credibility that comes with my position, and, consequently, certain changes are affected more readily as the structure allows the social work department to report at a high level in the institution with a significant amount of autonomy and flexibility in decision making.

On the other side of the ledger, the social work department does not get 100% of my time and attention. This inevitably means that certain operational issues and program development do not get attended to as carefully as they might with the full time attention and energy of a director. Similarly, from time to time social work staff perceive that not only are my interest and attention divided, leaving them with what feels like a part time administrator, but also that I have relinquished my social work identity and become a "business woman." Some view this as giving up social work ethics and values. From a practical point of view, while maintaining the dual responsibilities of social work director or administrator, it is essential to have a talented deputy upon whom one can rely totally, and a strong management team in the department of social work to carry out the operational and programmatic components in a maximally effective way.

CAREER EVOLUTION

To return to my initial comment about the relationship of my career evolution and societal changes, I feel compelled to say that my attitudes and approach to career advancement did not begin when I became a director of social work. To look at my evolution, I find myself going back to my entry to the profession and a set of plans and circumstances not dissimilar to those of many entering the profession at the time when I trained: my main interest was clinical social work. I saw my career as being one combining institution-based and private practice. My image of my life included being at home full time for a period of time, raising a family and following a traditional path well laid out before me by many women, including my mother. Apparently, lurking in the deeper recesses of my mind, however, were ambitions and goals fostered by my family during my adolescence. These lay dormant until a later time in my life. As I worked, and as the women's movement had an impact on nearly every corner of American life, the possibility of other opportunities became clear to me as years went on. Not only was there increased social acceptability of working and raising children at the same time, but the emerging possibility of selecting career options that involved a higher degree of assertiveness, risk, ambition, competition and aggression was both more externally acceptable and more personally acceptable to me

Some of the key components of skilled clinical practice left me unsatisfied. A passive position, a constant listening mode, and endless patience were not enough for me. I needed time in my work day where I could make decisions, move quickly, make things happen, be active and influence patient care more globally. My initial experiences with hospital management led me to believe that administration could gratify certain personal needs that clinical practice could not.

As my experience in management increased, I came to see that quality administration could evolve from a blend of characteristics normally associated with being a traditional clinical social worker and those of a traditional manager. The ability to translate certain aspects of the social work approach into health care administration is essential.

Integrating Social Work Competencies into Health Care Administration

Probably the most significant skill that social workers can bring to health care administration is their facility in interpersonal relationships—the ability to understand the needs and behaviors of others and to respond to the latent as well as the manifest content of communications. It is a cliché to remind people that organizations are composed of people, and good administrators are those who know how to respond to other individuals' agendas and to motivate others to carry out one's own agenda.

Adopting a different jargon, this means that social workers are—or can be—specialists in systems and organizational behavior. Health care institutions, particularly hospitals, are among the most complex institutions in our society. They seldom have the classic pyramidal structure of the corporation but rather have many competing constituencies, such as physicians, unions, and a wide range of employees from the highly skilled and technical to the unskilled. Health care institutions also contend with a multitude of outside influences including local, state and federal regulation, and a coterie of accrediting bodies. Consequently, affecting change or for that matter even getting anything done in a hospital can often be complex and difficult. Both through their training and way of thinking, social workers understand how to negotiate the hospital system. This skill, which is no more than a different way of looking at basic clinical skills, may range from covertly assisting with the group process in a meeting of administrators or understanding the politics of the institution in terms of how to achieve a controversial end.

The clinician's way of thinking, using latent content to understand the process, can be extremely helpful for effective functioning as an administrator particularly in as complex a setting as health care. The skill of converting the clinical interpretation to the well placed comment at the right time is useful. Understanding the importance of listening to people and working through issues is a clinical skill replicable and essential to administration. The capacity for empathy, the touchstone of clinical social work, is valuable in an administrator.

Another social work skill of great use in health care administration is the profession's comprehensive understanding of social policy. Public policy concerns impinge upon every corner of health care and the social worker's social policy knowledge base is increasingly helpful in the current climate of health care. It is not unusual for managers in health care settings, as anywhere else, to have a somewhat myopic view of their world with boundaries set by the walls of their institutions, let alone by a profession or guild. An understanding of the broadest context of health and social welfare policy may be exploited by the social work administrator to assist top management in fulfilling its goals and objectives. Such knowledge also aids in advocating for the priorities of social workers in health care.

On the other hand, some of the very skills that make a good clinician do *not* make a good administrator. For example, the tendency to encourage the clinician's passivity, sense of timelessness and endless patience are less appropriate qualities for an administrator. Consequently, the transition from clinician to administrator must involve a change in a social worker's style.

Traditionally, promotional opportunities in social work have been available only through movement into administrative positions within or outside of social service departments. This results inevitably in clinically skilled social workers becoming administrators because of their success as clinicians. While career development for social workers is not the issue at hand, those clinicians desirous of increasing their earnings and gaining additional prestige in their work may feel compelled to move into management. Such individuals may not successfully achieve the needed transition in style and work values. The new manager must learn to exercise authority in a different way with subordinates than with clients. He or she must have as a priority primarily the institution which serves clients, while the clinician's priority is the individual client.

As noted above, this move from clinician to administrator demands changes in perception, identifications, loyalty and values (Scurfield, 1981). When the social worker does not make these shifts in style and work values, quality of work as well as job satisfaction may suffer.

From Staff Social Worker to Senior Management; One Person's Transition

My transition was gradual and involved societal and cultural changes as well as intrapsychic changes. The early years of my career were comfortably passed following the traditional clinical social work devel-

opmental paths, from clinician to supervisor, teacher and private practi
tioner.

As I found myself evolving in a traditional social work career, I also
became increasingly in touch with a variety of personal motivations.
found myself more ambitious than I had realized, more interested in
gaining power, influence and authority, and more invigorated by making
an impact on issues larger than individual patient issues. Additionally,
my interests led me beyond clinical practice to an awakened passion
about social justice. My increasing awareness of a host of motivations,
including heightened consciousness of strivings for success, led me to
aggressively seek the directorship of social work of a large department
some seven years after graduating from social work school. Holding that
position gratified many of my interests and ambitions and clarified for me
that my career goals would continue to be in management rather than in
clinical practice, research or teaching. I found myself feeling competent
as a manager, and I enjoyed the dynamics of administration. I never had
any doubts that management satisfied certain of my fundamental strivings
and wishes.

After five years or so as director of social work, I once again became
aware of wanting more: more power, more influence, more economic
reward, and more potential impact on more programs. Again my response
was to seek out other opportunities aggressively. Because I had gained
credibility with top management, after a period of time other responsibilities were gradually made available to me. I did not immediately
acquire the whole set of responsibilities I now carry outside social work
nor did I immediately acquire an administrative title. This was an
incremental process, fought for every step of the way.

There is a critical component that runs through my personal transition
that assists me in understanding my motivations, and this is the issue of
mentoring. A mentoring relationship has been described as " . . . strong
emotional interchange between an older and younger person, where the
younger person feels encouraged to directly challenge the older person's
ideas and the older person has enough confidence to take it" (*Harvard
Business Review, 1978*). Mentoring is a concept that we as social workers
understand as it clearly has psychological roots in the process of
identification. My first mentor was my father, a social work executive,
and I can now trace my own development and administrative successes to
his influence. My explorations of my development reveal to me the
impact of my father, who was successful, ambitious, and highly
motivated; he had an exceptionally effective style as an executive and as
a leader. My father implicitly encouraged me to be like him and to take
on his ambitions and competitive strivings as well as his passions about
social justice. It was my father who taught me how to give a speech, how
to run a meeting and how to lead an organization. Whether it was editing

his speeches as an adolescent or watching him in operation, he taught me and I learned. While I was not consciously aware of my identifications as I was growing up, my personal growth and development allowed me to see that I could take his mentoring and positive ways without relinquishing other strivings, such as being a wife and mother.

My transition into health care administration was also aided immeasurably by other mentors, including a physician who headed a unit in which I worked and another physician who is president of my hospital.

As I indicated earlier, a key in this transition was my increasing awareness that because of social change, a woman now had "permission" concomitantly to have children, be feminine, and vigorously pursue career ambitions. This societal liberation was particularly important to me and assisted in mitigating my guilt about not being at home full time caring for children as my mother had.

There have been positive and negatives about my career advancement and both sides ought to be explored.

Positives and Negatives of Health Care Administration for the Social Worker

For the hospital social worker, moving from an unambiguous identity to a broader one is a novelty for both colleagues of other disciplines as well as for social work colleagues. Precedent setting brings with it pain and excitement. I found my advancement was regarded with suspicion by social work and nonsocial work colleagues alike. Hospital colleagues sometimes responded with jealousy and competitive feeling. Many denied that I had actually advanced and persisted in regarding my position exclusively as the management of the social work function despite any evidence to the contrary. Others devalued and denigrated administrative career advancement. I would have expected more social work colleagues outside my hospital to regard such advancement as potentially opening possibilities for them, however, in actuality, the response was highly ambivalent.

Social work staff also responded ambivalently to my advancement. On one hand, many saw it as an indication of greater career opportunities and precedent setting for them as social workers. Others saw the promotions as increasing the power and credibility of the social work function in the hospital. At the same time, some social workers expressed concern about my "abandonment" of the profession and presumed change in professional identity. Despite my insistence that I was still a social worker, many social workers saw me as moving into "business." This feeling was accompanied by a worry that the social work department had less of my time, interest and concern. Staff believed that I had outgrown them, which did, in fact, have a kernel of truth to it. Such issues should be dealt with as openly and honestly as is possible. Moreover, one also can demonstrate the use of the new position in the organization to advocate for social work interests.

As social workers become administrators, the change in role often brings conflicts, and of particular importance among them are ethical ones. As a social worker or even a social work director, the relatively unambiguous role is advocacy for the patient. It is expected in the health care setting and to some extent accepted that the director of social work may balance the institution's tendency to be concerned about its more narrowly defined self interest. In an administrative position, however, it is not as easy to take on this role. I have found myself at times being the "conscience" of the institution and while this has positive aspects, it also has negatives. It is obviously helpful for any individuals at a high level to be attentive to issues related to ethics. At the same time, the image of "professional conscience" or "do-gooder" can be an impediment. We know what people may do when they do not like the directives of their "conscience"; they may get rid of them.

I do not believe the social worker in the hospital ought to take the role of the "bleeding heart liberal." Social work does not necessarily have a monopoly on caring, and it is presumptuous to assume this. On the other hand, if we do not react with the patient's viewpoint when we participate in decision making about issues about which we have ethical concerns, we have our own consciences to reckon with. I have certainly confronted these dilemmas around discussions of free care dollar allocations or marketing and have not always been at peace with my role in these discussions. I do not have an answer to how one comes to terms with this. Such significant problems merit further exploration and recognition as social workers become health care administrators. If not adequately dealt with, excessive guilt and self doubt can result.

There is ample opportunity for self doubt when one moves into these new roles. Firstly, there are certain basic management skills needed that most social workers have not formally learned in graduate education. Probably the most important of these is financial management. While departmental management provides experience in budgeting and statistical reporting, senior administrative positions demand a more sophisticated and in-depth understanding of cost accounting, reimbusement, data processing and productivity formulae. In order to handle my work, I pursued, with the support of the hospital, several executive training courses.

Though I am sure it would be helpful, I have not felt strongly the need to get a masters degree in business administration. I recognize my weaknesses and have encouraged the hospital to use me in those areas to which I bring competence. For example, the hospital would do better to use others for sophisticated financial management or computerization initiatives. My skills lie in program planning, problem-solving, organizational change, and operations.

Fortunately, there is a congruence between my view of my strengths and top management's needs and views of my strengths. I think my experience can be generalized; it may not be necessary for social workers to obtain additional degrees. The skills of the social work profession in organizational change and in understanding the dynamics of systems are valuable assets to management. The clinician's emphasis on self awareness and introspection leads to better management. As the social worker advances he or she can retain the ability to listen, understand and look inward.

BEING A WOMAN HEALTH CARE ADMINISTRATOR

There are many critical issues for all social work administrators in health care settings, but there are specific and difficult ones for the woman hospital administrator. While 80% of the work force in hospitals is female, only 12% of hospital administrators are female. Hospital administration has offered limited growth opportunities for women, perhaps because of anachronistic attitudes of some physicians and trustees about women's roles. This is curious when one considers that hospitals used to be run by nurses and nuns. Classic female attributes such as caring, sensitivity, and the valuation of service to others are especially meaningful in a hospital (Friedman, 1980). Moreover, the administrative positions in hospitals that women have achieved so far are largely staff roles such as planning and public relations rather than operational, line management positions. The paucity of role models and precedence has made it even harder for women to advance administratively (Appelbaum, 1975). Advancement may occur more readily in the corporate world than the hospital.

Therefore, opportunities have been somewhat limited for women social workers to advance into management. Perhaps conflicts between traditional feminine self image and the image of administrators have deterred social workers from pursuing management positions. Those women social workers who do move into administrative positions seem to have more self esteem, more risk-taking ability and higher aspirations than others (Munson, 1982).

It is reasonable to conclude that the advancement of the women social worker into hospital administration is not an easy move. If the social worker has had the good fortune to be protected from sexism or sex role stereotyping in her traditional professional functions, she may be in for a rude awakening as an administrator. She may be surprised when she is automatically regarded as less ambitious, more emotional, more dependent, and less invested in her job than her male colleagues. The absence of role models only exacerbates this situation.

Women social work administrators may be unprepared for contending with an old boy network that is likely to be closed to them. Initially, they may think that their empathy, helpfulness, understanding and intuitive skills will be sufficient to evoke acceptance. They may not.

Women social work administrators need to be prepared to deal with the same kinds of issues that women frequently confront in all executive positions. Among these are salary equity concerns, acceptance of assertiveness and decisiveness, and at minimum, being listened to and respected. The process of acceptance and change may be difficult and slow with administrative colleagues, physicians and perhaps trustees. Proving one's competence may take longer, and more ability may be required than is of men. The woman social work administrator will undoubtedly find the process of acceptance or rejection and valuation or denigration to be complicated, confusing, and enervating. In the face of such dilemmas, the tendency is to withdraw and become fearful. If the individual is afraid of power and competition, fearful of earning too much money, or of being aggressive and assertive, debilitating conflict can result. In addition to the absence of role models, it is also unfortunate that few networks exist to assist women in handling these issues effectively.

CONCLUSIONS

While my own career development and advancement has been related to a set of complex personal factors, there are messages in my development that may have relevance for others. Clearly, there are opportunities in health care administration for social workers. Social work training is sufficiently generic to prepare individuals for a whole host of career options. Social work graduate education offers much in the way of useful preparation for administration. I do not feel it is essential to obtain additional graduate education, but rather to build on acquired skills and knowledge. Hopefully, social workers will be encouraged to take risks and pursue new, maybe unconventional career directions aggressively.

But being prepared and being qualified is only half the battle. Top administrators do not usually come to you and say, ''Would you like to share some of my power?'' Social workers who want to become administrators in health care settings, and to succeed in these roles, must become clear about what it is they want and take active steps in the direction of self-promotion in all senses of the word.

Ideally, the social worker trying to move into administrative positions should not have to stand alone. The profession has the opportunity and responsibility to prepare social workers for health care administration

ırough increased education and network development around the dilem-
ıas and learning needs I have delineated. Assistance needs to be
vailable to sort out ethical dilemmas, to explore specific issues for
ʻomen administrators, to explain and work through staff and colleagues'
ɛsponses to career advancement, and to enlarge the knowledge base for
ıch social workers.

The advancement of social workers into health care administration
ffers not only personal benefits to those individuals involved, but also
roadens the parameters and horizons of the social work field, thereby
ɛtting a positive precedent. Most importantly, it brings social work
ıeory, values, knowledge and skills into the highest level of decision
ıaking in health care settings, with the potential of influencing both
atient care, and the way in which health care institutions are managed.
ʻhus, such advancement offers the social work profession a significant
pportunity to have a positive influence on the delivery of quality health
are.

REFERENCES

ppelbaum, Alan L., 1975. "Women in Health Care Administration." *Hospitals, Journal of the American Hospital Association*, August 16, pp. 52–59.
riedman, Emily, 1980. "Women CEOS: They're Good for the Field But Is It Good for Them?" *Hospitals, Journal of the American Hospital Association*, February 1, pp. 45–48.
ʻarvard Business Review*, 1978. "Everyone Who Makes It Has A Mentor, Interview with F.J. Lunding, G.L. Clements and D.S. Perkins." July–August, pp. 89–101.
lunson, Carlton E., 1982. "Perceptions of Female Social Workers Toward Administrative Positions." *Social Casework*, 63(1), January, pp. 54–59.
curfield, Raymond, M., 1981. "Clinician to Administration: Difficult Role Transition?" *Social Work*, 26(6), November, pp. 495–501.

CHAPTER III

Social Worker
to Hospital Administrator

Steven J. Goe, MSW

For the past three years my role has been the Vice-President of Administration at Daniel Freeman Memorial Hospital[*], a 403 bed non-profit hospital near the Los Angeles Airport in Inglewood, California. One of thirteen hospitals supported by the Sisters of St. Joseph of Carondelet, Daniel Freeman is part of a two-hospital medical center prominent in rehabilitation, trauma and emergency medicine, and cardiology.

Reporting to the Executive Vice-President of the hospital corporation, my role as Vice-President of Administration is essentially that of the Chief Operating Office of the hospital. Reporting to me are the following administrative heads:

- Associate Administrator for Professional Services
- Associate Administrator for Rehabilitation Services
- Assistant Administrator for Support Services
- Assistant Administrator for DRG and Contract Programs
- as well as some directors of new product lines such as home health, the trauma center, transportation and others.

Nursing and finance departments report to their own respective vice-presidents. Thus, three vice-presidents (administration, nursing and finance) are responsible for the management of the hospital.

The Director of the Social Work Department is primarily accountable to the Associate Administrator for Rehabilitation Services. I use "prima-

Mr. Goe is now Administrator, Scripps Memorial Hospital, Encinitas, California 92020.

rily'' because the department has diversified to include some for-profit product lines which are responsible through the director to managers in the respective for-profit companies or foundation. Through these administrative heads I am ultimately accountable for the social work programs.

My movement into administration was not expected or planned. The primary reason I believe hospital administration sought me out was because of my activity in marketing and planning. Although "marketing" as such was not in vogue, the institution had the vision to see that the development of alternative health care delivery methods and new "product lines" was the key to their survival in the competitive future. If there was one most important social work skill that contributed to my movement in the organization, it was the ability to recognize the wants and needs of our patients and other customers.

TRANSITION

After receiving my MSW, I worked for a few years as a social worker in a health clinic and on a physical rehabilitation unit in an acute hospital. I started my career at Daniel Freeman Memorial Hospital over 10 years ago, as the only social worker in the hospital. My immediate priority was to service the basic social work needs of the existing units and clinics. This was accomplished through formal channels of proposal writing and demonstration studies but more effectively through bargaining and negotiation. Within a few years, when there was sufficient social work staffing to meet the immediate needs of the institution, my goals then centered around developing new services and programs to serve the needs and wants of our patients, physicians, community and hospital administration. As I developed new programs, it became necessary to decide how these programs would report administratively. Initially, such programs as employee assistance, contracting social work services to other hospitals and physician offices, and industrial treatment programs could be managed within the social work department. As new programs were developed, a transition in administrative relationships had to evolve. Grants which I obtained created new programs in such areas as: transportation for disabled and elderly, attendant training for homebound elderly, a community resource and advocacy center for the disabled, and an early screening and treatment program for developmentally high risk infants. Although these programs were developed under the social work department and had obvious strong social work involvement, the number of programs and their managers grew to the point that they required their own administrative head or else face being dispersed administratively throughout the organization. In order to maintain the integrity of the programs, I assumed the role of administrative assistant under rehabilitation. A new director of social work was recruited and reported to me. As I demonstrated the ability to operate these programs and to develop new services, particularly in rehabilitation, my role evolved to that of assistant, and then associate administrator with increased departmental and programatic responsibilities.

Part of my new role involved the development of consulting services in rehabilitation to other hospitals. This activity led to the development of a for-profit company which, along with several other trends, led to the restructuring of our organization to include for-profit companies, a foundation, a holding company and a management division. My vice-president at the time was promoted to executive director of the for-profit company. At the same time, the administrator of the hospital assumed executive roles in the new companies. A new role was created for a vice-president of administration to accommodate the administrator's move into involvement in the other companies. I was asked to step into this role at that time.

Members of the Board of Directors were aware of the fact that I had no formal training in hospital administration, business administration or finance. They stated their view at that time, that the talents I possessed most relevant for the position were strong management skills and leadership, but most importantly, creativity and vision, good listening and communication skills and positive relationships with all levels of personnel in the facility. The concensus was that these skills could not always be found in an MHA or MBA background.

LACK OF FORMAL ADMINISTRATIVE SKILLS

My transition to administration did not involve any formal training in administration or finance. The technical skills needed for operational decisions, such as accounting/finance, I have learned on the job. This "deficit" has never been a problem except initially, when I was challenged by colleagues in finance or by subordinates with MBAs or MHAs who wanted to test my skill base. I made a point of seeking out all answers to my accounting or financial questions. I found a mentor in my former administrative head whom I was able to trust with my most basic questions. I was safe to ask him for answers that would have made me feel threatened publically. I struggled until I understood financial statements and cost reports, and could discuss these reports knowledgeably at meetings. Most importantly, I gathered subordinates who were talented in these areas and whom I could trust.

My opinion is that my lack of formal administration or financial training was never a hindrance to my role. Frankly, I am not sure that another advanced degree would have better prepared me. It was my social work skills applied in a new way in new situations that were helping me to adapt and become successful. Technical "administrative" skills which I could learn "on the job" served to augment and support my professional skills.

SOCIAL WORK SKILLS

Marketing

I feel strongly that the foundation of my transition was built on marketing and planning skills. Marketing is not new to social work, the label applies to a group of basic social work skills: assessment and interviewing, program development and community organization. Marketing in its generic sense is defined as a process to develop new products (services) that will meet the wants of your customers. The process includes:

1. surveying the needs and wants of your customers;
2. developing a product or service that will meet the wants;
3. promoting the product to your customer;
4. evaluating the effectiveness of the product in meeting the need; and
5. refining the product and repromoting it.

These are skills endemic to social work training. No other professional in the hospital is better equipped with the skills in needs assessment nor better informed on the wants and needs of its community. Social workers are trained to identify through interviews the needs, wants and problems of our individual clients. We develop goals to meet these needs. When the service does not exist to meet the need, we are creative in our approaches to finding one that does, or in designing such a resource. At another level, social work administrators take this process to a macro level to develop a program or service that will meet the needs of an identified group of clients. This can be accomplished through an organized, documented effort using consumer studies and design, or through community organization tools.

I believe that the social work training in graduate school most relevant to my current role was in community organization. The skills learned in recognizing and working with power structures in organizations and communities have been vital. Tactics and strategies for bringing about social change were transferred to an institutional framework. To bring about change in my organization I needed to apply the principles of first understanding the institution, its needs, its mission, its purpose and its power structure. The key to my success in developing new programs and services was in understanding how social change priorities fit on a spectrum of priorities for the hospital; and how they could be presented as compatible and mutually supportive (Rosenberg and Weissman, 1981).

An example of this was the development of our employee assistance program. The social work department identified as a top priority the need to develop employee assistance services to our hospital employees. Administration reviewed our proposals and agreed it was a need but not a priority, so could not earmark funds at that time. The hospital's priority was, however, to develop new products for the industrial market. Understanding this priority, we developed an EAP package and promoted it to industrial clients. When several contracts were signed, we could demonstrate their accrual of sufficient capital to initiate our own in-house service. This strategy of "combining missions" was successful in developing profitable new markets for the hospital but, more importantly, in serving many unmet social work needs that certainly would have remained unserved.

A major adjustment I have had to make moving into administration, however, is in the adaption of these community organization skills. As a social worker and then as a social work department director, I could use these tactics relatively unnoticed. Whether this is a learned social work skill or selective social work trait, successful social workers are willing to take risks. Manipulation, bargaining and negotiation were strategies I could use freely throughout the organization to bring about change. Often new services or changes were initiated without the knowledge or formal approval of administration. As an administrator now, however, each decision I make is highly exposed and open to the scrutiny of other executives and the Board. Until I fully adapt these strategies to my new level, I continue to use my informal networks in the institution to facilitate changes that would be too cumbersome or political through a formal process.

Popple (1984) speaks to negotiation as a critical skill in social work administration. In fact, according to his survey, administrators engage in negotiation up to twenty-six percent of their time. Negotiation is not taught formally as a skill in social work education but is part of community organization and organizational theory. I submit that this is such a valuable skill that it needs separate attention in social work training. Social workers as administrators have transferred these skills in processes appropriate to their organizational settings.

Assessment and Interviewing

Psycho-social assessment skills learned in graduate school have been important tools in the Board Room as well as in brief administrative update meetings. Now an automatic process, I formulate a "brief psycho-social assessment" on all the players in a room when I walk into a meeting. I quickly assess their needs and wants and based on these findings determine my course of approach in the meeting. These skills along with my social

work intuition have given me an advantage over my administrative colleagues in problem solving and managing crisis situations.

Group Process

Similarly, my social work training in group process and dynamics has
been critical to my conduct of meetings, assignment of task forces as well
as my role of group member. I find it interesting to go off on "executive
retreats" to learn skills in group leadership which were basic to my
graduate training. My ability to form a group, select its members, define
its purpose and goals, facilitate its process and lead it to a successful
conclusion, I attribute directly to my graduate group training. Obviously
the majority of groups I am now involved with are short-termed, task
specific committees.

Communication/Listening

An additional social work skill important to my administrative role is
listening and communication. Good communication skills are a key
ingredient to leadership. Administrators who are good leaders listen to
their staff. This enables then, to know how and where to lead them. More
importantly, good listening puts me in touch with the needs and wants of
their divisions. It is an art which I find evident in few of my colleagues
who have had only formal administrative training.

ADJUSTMENT TO MY NEW ROLE

Throughout the first year of my new role I experienced a tremendous
sense of isolation and lack of identity. This is apparently typical to social
workers who take on administrative careers, particularly clinicians who
move into supervisor or manager roles (Kugal and Riggs, 1981;
Holloway, 1980). However, the literature relates to social workers who
administer clinical departments within a clinical environment, in other
words, social work administrators. I feel my transition was more notable
in that I needed to assume a whole new role and identity, a new
profession for which I had no formal training.

I felt tremendously alienated. I was not yet an administrator, and I was
no longer a social worker. My "clinical-administrative" model was no
longer an appropriate one (Scurfield,1981). I found it difficult to identify
with other administrators both socially and professionally. I felt out of
place with them and insecure about my skills in interacting with them. I
missed the collaborative fellowship of social work professional networks.

It took a long time before I was able to overcome this insecurity and establish an identity of my own; as a hospital administrator who is also a social worker. I acquired the skills necessary to identify myself as a hospital administrator, but I have also appreciated the contribution of my social work skills to my administrative style and success. I no longer struggle with "who am I" professionally and the insecurities of not feeling complete in either profession. I am secure in the fact that my mixture of skills and talents is a unique and successful blend. Another difficulty I experienced in moving from social work director to administrator was in developing a more direct, decisive management style. Clinically I was trained in the dynamic, indirect techniques. I was rewarded in seeing growth in my social work supervisees through this approach.

There is a place for this technique in executive management, however. The effective leader takes a direct approach to his decision making. Leaders make the right decision at the right time. Effective leaders are able to take a stand that may not be popular and stand by it when they know it represents the best course of action. This often means not taking the luxury of facilitating this decision in others through indirect approaches. However, analytical training has continued to pay-off in helping me to follow a logical course of action for making the right decision and knowing when to involve others in the decision-making process.

QUALITIES OF ADMINISTRATORS

Effective administrators all possess three basis skills: *technical, human, conceptual* (Katz, 1978). The technical involves specialized knowledge, analytical ability within that specialty, and the facility to use the tools and techniques of that specialty. In my transition into hospital administration I gained the specialized knowledge of my new profession "in the field" and through independent study of journals and texts. I brought with me the analytical ability and facility to use the tools.

The human skill is the administrator's ability to work effectively as a group member and to build a cooperative effort within his team. My social work training in human behavior, psycho dynamic work with individuals and groups prepared me in this area more than any graduate program in hospital administration or business administration could have.

The third skill, conceptual, includes the ability to envision the institution as a whole and to understand how different functions interact with each other. Although I took a graduate social work course in organization theory, my knowledge foundation comes from social systems theory.

There seems to be a trend in the market place today to hire

administrators who come from the business sector with MBAs from prestigious business schools. Many hospitals now seem to prefer MBA over MHAs, particularly in the for-profit sector. It is possible from what we know of effective administration that this trend could have a backlash that will be felt all the way into the community. Longest (1978) discusse the critical importance of environmental assessment and the impact of those changes on the operation of the hospital. He points out that operational strategies must be formulated on knowledge of demography epidemiology and resource gaps in the community. The administrator of the future will need to be highly responsive to the community, a consumers begin to choose their providers on factors other than cost.

CONCLUSIONS

The literature is replete with studies of the transition from clinician to supervisor or clinic administrator. Until this book there were no refer- ences to the transition from clinical director to hospital executive. This movement involved two major changes: (1) assuming a new profession from social worker to administrator, with all its own skills and knowl- edge; and (2) moving into a new setting, from a social work to health care business identity. To understand this concept I have turned to literature on (1) the adjustment of changing professions, (2) the transition from clinician to supervisor, (3) the fundamentals of executive management and (4) the fundamentals of hospital administration.

When one studies the keys to executive management and leadership, one can create a list of specific technical skills required of that profession. To be such an executive in health care requires all of those skills, but in addition, a higher level of understanding of social systems and environ- mental interactions. Hospital administrators, unlike most executives of non-health industries, must apply management principles to the ultimate "high touch" business. Our products are not widgets but health and human services. Our employees have made a special life commitment to serving human needs. Our community expects that their needs and wants will be met by this institution. To manage and lead this kind of organization effectively requires very special skills: social work skills. My career path was such that I learned the social work skills first, and then the business skills. All hospital administrators continue to learn "hospital administration" skills as the nature of the business is changing rapidly. There is no longer one set of skills that a hospital administrator possesses that will make and keep him successful. Effective administra- tors are going through transitions themselves with their institutions and their communities. Marketing, product-line management, cost accounting, data base management, for example, are all new or renewed concepts for health care executives.

There is no emerald city that grants all the skill, knowledge, courage and heart needed to be a hospital administrator. They consist of a blend of skills and knowledge. Many skills of social work are part of this blend. These skills are what separate a hospital administrator from other business executives. A social work director must see what he has in common with his administrator. Their missions are not dissimilar, their priorities may be. An effective social work director must understand these similarities, seek common ground and not operate the department as a separate entity in a host environment. At that point he will see the whole hospital as a social work agency.

REFERENCES

Holloway, Stephen. "Up the Hierarchy: From Clinician to Administrator," *Administration in Social Work*, 4(Winter, 1980), 1–14.
Katz, Robert L. "Skills of an Effective Administrator," *Paths Toward Personal Progress: Leaders are Made, Not Born*, 1978, Harvard Business Review, Boston.
Kugal, Linda and Riggs, Thomas. "Practitioner to Administrator," *Social Casework: The Journal of Contemporary Social Work*, 62(April, 1981), 241–244.
Longest, Jr., Beaufort, B. "The Contemporary Hospital Chief Executive Officer," *Health Care Management*, Spring, 1978, 43–53.
Popple, Philip. "Negotiation: A Critical Skill for Social Work Administrators," *Administration in Social Work*, 8(Summer, 1984), 1–11.
Rosenberg, Gary and Weissman, Andrew. "Marketing Social Services in Health Care Facilities," *Health and Social Work*, 6(August, 1981), 13–20.
Scurfield, Raymond Monsour. "Clinician to Administrator: Difficult Role Transition?" *Social Work*, (November, 1981), 495–501.

CHAPTER IV

Pathway to Administration

Marybeth Flower, LCSW

CURRENT POSITION

I am the Assistant Administrator of the Division of Education at Pacific Presbyterian Medical Center, a teaching hospital which began as the West's first medical school in the late nineteenth century. Between 1908 and 1959 it was the site of Stanford University's Medical School and Hospital. In 1959, Stanford moved the medical school and hospital to its main campus in Palo Alto. Seventy-five percent of the faculty chose not to relocate but to remain at Pacific Presbyterian. Since Stanford's departure, the Center has continued to place a strong emphasis on its education function and consistently has made resources available for education programs.

As Assistant Administrator, I have direct reporting responsibility to a physician who reports directly to the President of the Medical Center, also a physician. I have administrative responsibility for eleven programs:

1. Graduate Medical Education
2. Continuing Education
3. Patient Education
4. Health Sciences Library
5. Community Education
6. Safety Training
7. Outreach Education
8. Audio-Teleconferencing
9. Micro-Surgery Training Laboratory
10. Media Services
11. Video Teleconferencing

The Division of Education is a separate division whose annual budget is $3,000,000. It provides service to a variety of groups: the board of trustees, medical staff, house staff, allied health professionals, business and industry, the employees and the community.

My role is to oversee the management of these eleven programs, to conduct long range planning for the division, identify centerwide educational needs and to ensure that the department managers I supervise have adequate resources to operate their departments with quality and efficiency. In addition, the division is embarking on several entrepreneurial projects which include the development of a for-profit slide making service and a revenue producing teleconferencing service. One of the planned teleconferencing projects involves fund-raising. This has been an interesting skill to learn as asking for money from individuals in the community is a departure from my social work experience. It has required some rethinking on my part to be comfortable in the asking instead of the giving side of the equation. Nonetheless, developing these new for-profit services and fund-raising skills is exciting. When the project is completed, I will have a new set of skills that will enhance my existing social work and administrative skills.

TRANSITION

The actual transition into administration was initiated by me. I was working in another community hospital that was characterized by a formal communication style. Department heads, for the most part, used surnames, not first names. The hospital had been managed for thirty-three years by a strong, formal leader who retired two weeks after my employment as Director of Social Service. The new chief executive officer was a young, dynamic man who wanted to modernize the hospital's mission and outlook. One day, obviously disappointed by a department head meeting that consisted of one-way communication from the top down, he asked me why department heads never spoke during these meetings. Sharing my assessment, I noted that he was a new administrator, had not yet gained the trust of the group, the meeting format did not encourage two-way communication, and he was following a strong, formal leader who had not encouraged two-way communication. Managers did not know what was expected of them and most of them had not been trained in management. I suggested that he consider the use of management training sessions with small groups of department heads, to begin to develop a more open, trusting atmosphere, to forge a management team and to help his department heads develop managerial skills.

Subsequent to this discussion, an assistant administrator and I developed a proposal to conduct an 8-week management training program for all department heads in groups of sixteen members or less. Six months later, the administrator asked if I still believed that I could run management training groups. I thought that I did not have content expertise in management training, but I knew group methods and could facilitate the group's processes. He agreed to hire a health care management training consultant, who taught me course content, how to write learning objectives and how to design educational programs.

The program was successful and within one and a half years the program had developed effective managers who displayed a team spirit that exceeded highest expectation. Although the administrator and I have since left the organization, most of the managers are still there. Their team spirit has remained high and they operate effectively under matrix style of management. Communication is open and there is now two-way communication at department head meetings.

As I began to have success with management training, I learned what were for me two new areas of health care education, that of health promotion and community health education. The hospital was constructing a new ambulatory care center. As one component of the marketing plan for this center I suggested that we send physicians, nurses, nutritionists and social workers out to the senior citizen hotels, boarding houses, and daycare programs to provide useful health education information and to inform them of the services available in the ambulatory care center. This program was followed by the development of ongoing health education programs at the hospital. At this point, I recommended that a Department of Education and Training be established. I was able to convince the hospital Chief Executive Officer that I could administer both the Social Work Department and the Education and Training Department, if an assistant director position was added to the social work table of organization. My title then became Administrative Director of Education, Training and Social Service. This position fell in a never-never land between department head and administration. I was not considered a hospital administrator, yet I was above the department head level. As I reflect back on this, I think it would have been important to have negotiated an administrator's position at that time.

Once the education department was established, I was able to expand programs to other areas. Within 18 months of developing the management training program, I had developed education programs for patients, employees, business and industry.

The transition to the next level of management came with a move to another hospital. The movement to administration was one that I planned, took risks to achieve and ultimately reached. It did not occur by happenstance. I was able to identify the areas where I needed to obtain and develop skills and knowledge, and then to demonstrate that I had effectively integrated them.

Why was I interested in moving into administration? It became apparent to me in my first job in a hospital that the social work director

was at the mercy of an administrator for access to resources. Th
administrator, the senior management team, and the board of trustee
determine the direction of the hospital and how departments ar
programs will be funded. I believed it was important to have decisic
making capabilities in the allocation of resources and that to gain th
capability it was necessary to move to the administrative level. Th
challenge of stretching myself to the next level was thrilling.

My current position does not include responsibility for the social wor
department. Ideally, I would have preferred to have maintained thi
responsibility. However, the corporate structure of the organization di
not permit for this since the Division of Education is a freestandin
division outside of the hospital structure of which the social wor
department is a component. I think we are only now beginning to tap th
rich resources social workers can bring to hospital systems of care and
would have wanted to be actively involved in helping to forward thei
increased utilization.

As I look back on the five years that have elapsed since I moved int
administration and relinquished responsibility for social work, I know i
has been and is a challenging and rewarding experience. Yet there ar
times when I miss the humanism that social workers bring to their work
My position requires that I speak "administratese" which translates int
a financial language rather than a human one. However, my social wor
skills enrich my work with my staff. Many social work groups invite m
to speak, occasions which keep me connected with my social work root
and the "human" side of health care.

I consider myself fortunate to have reached my current level withou
additional formal education being required. On an informal basis I sough
out numerous learning experiences. I worked intensively with the
consultant who trained me to conduct the management training programs
In addition, I attended numerous management training workshops and
read voraciously books on management, business and particularly marketing. Books by Drucker (1973), Kotler (1975), McDonald and Rubright (1981) and Spiro (1977) have been particularly helpful.

KNOWLEDGE, SKILLS, EDUCATION

I believe there are a number of social work skills that can be used in
health administration.

Start Where the Client Is

The client in health care administration can be the system, the
community, the physicians, or the employees. These groups can be
further divided into sub-groups or target markets. Ascertaining each

group's needs, wants and desires is essential. Social work skills are helpful in probing, questioning, clarifying and determining real needs. My social work training has been helpful in distinguishing between individual's stated and hidden agendas.

Study, Assessment and Treatment

The three phases of social casework; study, assessment and treatment are applicable to management problem solving. First, one studies the management problem and is able to differentiate the real problem from the perceived problem (diagnosis). This is similar to differentiating the symptom from the real problem in social work with individuals and groups. Once one understands the basic problem, a solution to the problem can be developed and implemented. This is similar to the development of a social work treatment plan. As in all clinical social work, frequently the plan needs to be altered. The practice of social casework has taught me the importance of thoroughly understanding the problem before jumping quickly to a treatment plan. The ability to study problems without immediately jumping to quick solutions is essential in management.

Facilitating Group Process

Understanding of groupwork theory and group facilitation is another useful skill in health care administration. A member of a health care administration team spends many hours each week in meetings. The knowledge of how to facilitate the process of meetings is helpful in keeping groups focused to the assigned task. With the success of Japanese Quality Circles and their importation to the United States, more health care organizations are implementing exact or modified versions of this structure. An increased emphasis is being placed on group process in decision making. I believe that this trend will continue as technology continues to develop rapidly. Today it is becoming increasingly more difficult for any one individual in an organization to have all the knowledge necessary to make key decisions. The knowledge of group process is helpful in understanding meetings. The communication patterns in meetings tell much about the organization, the person chairing the meeting and the individual members. The astute student of group process can use this information to function within the organization more effectively. I use what I learn at meetings to ascertain which projects, ideas and values different individuals support. This knowledge has been helpful when I have needed support for a new project, program or capital equipment since I know whom I can recruit successfully to help support my proposal or request. Such alliances are useful particularly with physicians who have power as clinicians who admit patients to the hospital.

Listening and Clarifying Skills

Business leaders recently have identified the need for their staffs to learn to listen more effectively. Courses and workshops designed to teach the art of listening are being offered across the country. Listening is a skill developed in casework and groupwork courses. When applied to health care management these same listening skills can be helpful in business communication. As I learned in graduate school "it is important to hear what the person is saying and what he is not saying." This axiom applies to all communication and is particularly helpful in health care administration.

Understanding Human Behavior

Knowledge of basic human needs and drives is helpful in understanding not only clients but all levels of hospital staff, those who report to you as well as your superiors and your clients. Understanding the basic human needs of employees can assist you in providing job satisfaction which increases their morale and productivity. Knowledge of non-verbal communication is essential for succeeding in management since the major portion of many messages is transmitted non-verbally rather than explicitly.

WHAT WAS LACKING

Not included in my social work education were some components that would have enhanced both my ability to manage a hospital social work department and to move into hospital administration. These components may have been lacking at the particular graduate school I attended and I do not know if these comments can be extrapolated to graduate curricula at other schools.

The Broad Picture

No emphasis was placed on the importance of looking at the environment and its impact on current and future programs. Nor was there content on how to read the environment and predict future trends effectively. The school I attended had a microcosmic view of the environment. A macrocosmic orientation would have been important in preparing me for a management position.

Strategy

Casework, groupwork and fieldwork courses taught me strategy in the context of how to intervene with patients and families in treatment plans. Strategy was not included in my social work administration courses. Strategy is important in my current position as an administrator. It is important that I think through what new programs I should develop and the impact they will have on my staff, other departments and other hospitals that are providing this service.

Budgeting

I do not recall ever discussing budgets in my social work administration courses. This was by far the hardest skill for me to learn as a new social work director. Budgeting remains the least favorite function in my current position, although during the past year I have learned a new appreciation for working with numbers.

Marketing

As a profession, we have not been effective in marketing ourselves. The profession is not viewed as having skills that are transferable to other fields. In general, it has been my personal observation that the field of social work is generally held in low esteem. In marketing terms we have an image problem which has affected the positioning of the social work profession within the job marketplace.

As a profession we need to learn to promote ourselves by educating employers, boards of trustees and the public at large about our skills and abilities. Until we learn to do this effectively, social workers will continue to find it difficult to move into positions of power and the salary levels of social workers will remain low.

Not only should social work schools teach us how to market the profession, they should also include basic marketing research techniques. As social workers, we are the advocates for the people we serve. In a period of limited resources and high competition, numbers speak. If we, as a profession, knew the basics of market research we could more effectively represent the populations we serve to the decision makers in our organizations and in our society.

CONCLUSION

Enhancing Administrative Potential

In pursuit of the early defined goal to move into hospital administration, I used a number of techniques and strategies on a fairly consistent basis.

Speak Their Language

In the course of their work, administrators have to work with and relate to a wide variety of individuals, each of whom have their own professional vernacular, unfamiliar to the administrator for the most part. Social work terms usually sound like jargon to the administrators. Since individuals who speak and discuss issues in familiar terms are more likely to be heard than those who use unfamiliar ones, it is important to avoid social work jargon and to use common verbal communication coinage.

Put Yourself in the Administrator's Shoes

Look at the organization through the eyes of your administrator. What are his problems and concerns? In what ways can you and your department actively help resolve problems, further the organization's interest and make its operation more effective?

See the Broad Picture

Be knowledgeable about your organization, its health care environment and the community in which it is situated. Are there opportunities for you and your department to take a leadership role in helping resolve problems?

Communicate Effectively

Learn to listen carefully. Use your perception skills to read nonverbal language. Develop assertive communications skills and effectively tell others about your department and its capabilities. Use in-house publications as a method of making your department more visible.

Unmet Needs

Identify some organizational needs and deficiencies. How can the social work department help to correct them?

Expand Your Department's Role

Move into new territory. Rather than wait for someone to ask or suggest that you or the department take on a new function, suggest the move yourself.

Know Your Department's Strengths

Have a good understanding of the strengths and weaknesses within your department. Be cognizant of your staff's specific skills and abilities. How can they be utilized to improve the organization and its services?

Help Your Peers and Subordinates

Help your colleagues. Be supportive of their endeavors. Help develop your subordinates. By helping others in the organization, you are helping the organization become a better institution.

Take Risks

Contrary to popular belief, opportunity usually does not knock on your door. Find opportunities in which to take professional risks. If you fail or falter, consider these learning experiences. Move on to carve out new opportunities for yourself and your department.

Never Rest on Your Laurels

Continue to grow and develop. Don't stop risking. Don't stop learning. The health care environment is ever changing. Continue to grow and develop in order to stay current.

When in connection with this book, I told a number of my business friends that I was trying to define what social work skills, theory and knowledge were helpful in movement from social work to health care administration, the universal response was laughter and "that's easy—none." I was surprised when a graduate social worker, successful as executive director of a residential treatment center for emotionally disturbed children, had the same response. Hospital administrators also had similar misconceptions about social workers and their skills. Indeed, one administrator suggested I delete Licensed Clinical Social Worker (LCSW) from my business card because people would view me as a social worker and not as a "competent administrator." I don't agree with their perception of social work. I think their negative view of social work is a result of social work's failure to market the profession effectively. Social workers have a negative image problem which needs correction and is correctable. I certainly found this to be so in my own career where I had direct experience of the fact that social work had much to contribute to the administration of health care programs and institutions.

REFERENCES

Drucker, P. *Management: Tasks, Responsibilities, Practices.* New York: Harper & Row, 1973.
Kotler, P. *Marketing for Nonprofit Organizations.* Englewood Cliffs, N.J.: Prentice-Hall, Inc., 1975.
McDonald, D. & Rubright, R. *Marketing Health and Human Services.* Rockville, Maryland: Aspen, 1981.
Spiro, H. *Finance for the Nonfinancial Manager.* New York: John Wiley & Sons, 1977.

CHAPTER V

The Social Worker as Leader

Karil S. Klingbeil, MSW

Increasingly, directors of social work departments in hospitals are assuming greater administrative responsibility and major administrative posts in health care settings. Two models seem to be emerging which have identifiable behaviors, traits and characteristics. One characterizes the social work director who continues in the position as director and is appointed to a position as either assistant or associate administrator of several units or departments in the hospital. Another model characterizes the social work director who vacates the social work department to assume an administrative role in a hospital or health care setting.

This chapter deals with the first model of social work directors who have broadened their administrative role in health care settings; and delineates the leadership qualities, skills and knowledge specific to this emerging management role.

BACKGROUND/SETTING

Harborview Medical Center is a 330 bed tertiary care teaching hospital of the University of Washington in Seattle. Founded in 1877, the hospital functioned as the county welfare facility caring for the medically indigent of King County. Although a major teaching hospital, this mission continued through the 1960s when the University of Washington contracted with King County to manage and operate the hospital. In the ensuing years, the County has played an important and more aggressive role in influencing the hospital's mission and in 1984 the Board of Trustees of Harborview Medical Center, appointed by the King County Executive, announced nine priority populations to be served by the hospital faculty and staff. These priority patients include persons incarcerated in the King County Jail; mentally ill patients, particularly those treated involuntarily; persons with sexually transmitted diseases; substance abusers; indigent patients without third party coverage; non-English speaking poor; trauma patients; burn patients; and those requiring specialized emergency care.

One of two primary teaching hospitals of the University of Washington Health Sciences, Harborview is a regional health care facility for the Pacific Northwest and Alaska. The Medical Center's comprehensive mission is to provide exemplary patient care, teaching, research and community service. The Northwest Regional Burn Center, Level I Emergency Trauma Center, Regional Epilepsy Center and a nationally recognized Sexual Assault Center are located at Harborview, in addition to the Medical Center's comprehensive inpatient services and more than 50 outpatient clinics which provide both primary and specialty care. Additionally, both Medic I, a mobile intensive coronary care program, and Airlift Northwest, a flying hospital unit, are operated out of Harborview.

SOCIAL WORK DEPARTMENT

In its early years, the Social Service Department in the county hospital was a branch of the local State Department of Social and Health Services. The primary role of staff was to determine patients' eligibility for various federal and state entitlement programs enabling access to medical care. During management contract negotiations with the University of Washington in 1967, the welfare office withdrew their staff and the Social Service Department, a professionally staffed, two-person unit emerged. I joined the Department as director in November, 1969, after seven years as clinical social worker, supervisor, program director and clinical faculty (School of Social Work) at University Hospital, another teaching facility of the University of Washington.

These were transition years for Harborview as it became a more comprehensive academic health care facility. New administrative staff and department heads were hired. Opportunities abounded in leadership, program development, community networking, coalition-building and for creative, innovative and daring program endeavors. Almost immediately, I changed the Department name to Social Work Department in an effort to emphasize its professional directions of psychosocial assessment, community resource management, discharge planning, and short-term psychotherapy. At the same time, the Volunteer Department, Chaplaincy Program and special Patient Care Funds were added to my administrative responsibilities. As the professional staff grew in numbers, the teaching, research, and community service missions became clearly articulated responsibilities and broadened the role of Social Work personnel, both in the hospital and in the community.

During this growth period (1970–1980) the Department expanded both internally and externally. Many social work staff were appointed to important hospital committees and boards. They also became experts in specialized practices and resource management thereby extending the boundaries of the hospital into the community. The Medicaid/Discharge Unit, Sexual Assault Center and Emergency Room Social Work Unit evolved as specialty programs enhancing the Department's professional expertise and ever-increasing credibility in the hospital, region and nation. Clearly, given the implication of the social mission of Harborview Medical Center described earlier, the Social Work Department has always played a major role in "administrative matters" including the political relationships with county and city governments. The mission of the hospital and the mission of the Social Work Department have been synonymous.

As the Department Director, I was instrumental in developing some of the specialized programs and in providing the leadership for others in the Department to develop programs on the cutting edge of clinical practice. As the success of these innovative ventures multiplied, hospital administration recognized the Social Work Department's contribution and leadership, and reached out to request my assistance and support in program efforts and other developments. Some innovations occurred internally within the Social Work Department whose members expanded their professional roles and responsibilities. Additionally, program development occurred outside the Department as individuals in the Department provided leadership in the hospital organization and policy setting arenas. For example, the Medicaid Application/Discharge Unit, the invention of the Social Work Department, was strongly supported and assisted by administration in concert with Harborview's mission. Specially trained staff were selected to deal with troubled patients and families, those in grief, those who were angry and hostile, those who were embarrassed and ashamed and those who otherwise might be considered at high risk and vulnerable. These key staff have continued to serve the patient/family in a holistic sense, thereby enhancing cooperation and compliance and maximizing reimbursement to the hospital. The Social Work Department continues to provide leadership in meeting patient need, the priorities of administration and the Department's goals and objectives by creating new opportunities to serve the population and developing cost effective solutions to acute care hospitalization. Recently, the Department participated with the Planning Office in contracting for special nursing home beds for those patients who require less than acute care, but who needed further rehabilitation beyond the hospital setting. This innovation decreased length of stay and addressed the patients needs while at the same time enabled the flow of emergency admissions for trauma patients, one of Harborview's primary mission populations.

The Social Work Department is comprised of eight administrative units and several distinct programs wtihin those units. They include the Executive Senior Staff Unit; the Emergency Room Social Work Unit; Medicine Unit; Medicaid Application/Discharge Unit; Psychiatry Unit; Surgical Unit; the Women and Children's Unit; and the Sexual Assault Center. Units are organized programmatically around service areas and comprise a continuity of care theme including inpatient and outpatient responsibility. (See Figure 1.)

SOCIAL WORK DIRECTOR AS ADMINISTRATOR

In August, 1981, I was appointed to a position as Acting Assistant Administrator of the hospital. This position was made permanent in 1984 and represented the first time in the University of Washington system that a social worker occupied an administrative position in the health science structure. Like the few similar colleagues around the country, the position carried with it the continuing role as Director of Social Work but added major responsibilities for several other programs and departments in the hospital with the title of Assistant Administrator for Ambulatory Care and Mental Health. The position is responsible for all fiscal, supervisory and administrative management for the outpatient clinics, specialty clinics and two outreach clinics, one in the historical Pioneer Square area (Skid

FIGURE 1

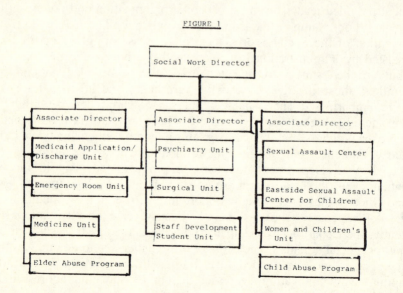

Road) and the other the Millionair Club Clinic, a multiservice agency
serving the "new poor" and indigent of the downtown area. Other
responsibilities include the Harborview Community Mental Health Center; Social Work Department, including its Sexual Assault Center,
Medicaid Application/Discharge Unit, Emergency Room Unit and other
program units described in Figure I; Patient Registration areas (both
Emergency Trauma Center and outpatient clinics); Involuntary Treatment
Program; Pastoral Care Department; Psychometric Testing Laboratory;
and Employee Health. Several additional programs and administrative
responsibilities include that of chairperson of patient welfare funds; of the
Hospital Discharge Planning, Health and Safety, and Hospital Policy
Manual Committees; administrative representative to the Hospital Infection Control, the Quality Assurance, the New Employee Orientation and
the Minority Affairs Committees. In addition, I represent the hospital in
several city-wide task forces and committees related to the street people
and the homeless population in Seattle; I am representative to the
community clinic coalitions and networks; and represent the hospital on
special committees such as the Seattle Police Department Task Force on
Harrassment and the Community Service Officers Advisory Group.

A new administrative effort for which I am responsible as its Executive
Director is the Harborview Center for the Study of Interpersonal
Violence. This center is part of the Social Work Department, Harborview
Community Mental Health Center, School of Social Work, and the
Department of Psychiatry and Behavioral Sciences. A major research
effort, the Center will bring together all types of research in interpersonal
violence, working closely with service programs throughout the city and
region. Figure 2 depicts my administrative responsibilities.

I am also a member of the Faculty at the University of Washington,
holding the positions of Assistant Professor in the School of Social Work
and adjunct Assistant Professor in the Department of Psychiatry and
Behavioral Sciences in the Medical School. Since 1984 the Faculty
position in the School of Social Work includes the role of Chair of the
Health Care Concentration. My particular Assistant Administrator position thus comprises a unique blend of academic as well as administrative
activities and responsibilities in the health care arena.

THE TRANSITION

Being an administrator has been a major goal since my graduate education in social work which was seasoned with intriguing managerial and
administrative coursework. Additionally, in the late 1960s, I took all the
academic courses at the University of Washington in the program for the
masters degree in public administration. I did not complete the thesis

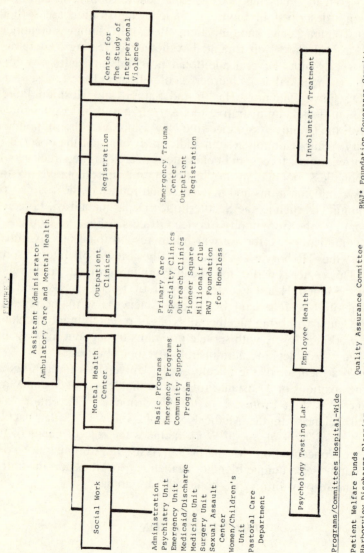

FIGURE

Assistant Administrator Ambulatory Care and Mental Health

Center for The Study of Interpersonal Violence

Social Work

- Administration
- Psychiatry Unit
- Emergency Unit
- Medicaid/Discharge
- Medicine Unit
- Surgery Unit
- Sexual Assault Center
- Women/Children's Unit
- Pastoral Care Department

Mental Health Center

- Basic Programs
- Emergency Programs
- Community Support Program

Outpatient Clinics

- Primary Care
- Specialty Clinics
- Outreach Clinics
- Pioneer Square
- Millionair Club
- RWJ Foundation for Homeless

Registration

- Emergency Trauma Center
- Outpatient Registration

Psychology Testing Lab

Employee Health

Involuntary Treatment

Programs/Committees Hospital-Wide

- Patient Welfare Funds
- Harborview Discharge Planning Committee
- Health and Safety Committee
- Infection Control Committee

- Quality Assurance Committee
- Policy Manual
- Employee Orientation
- Minority Affairs
- Ambulatory Care

RWJ* Foundation Goverance Committee
*(Robert Wood Johnson – Pew Memorial)
County/City of Seattle Committees
Seattle Police Department Committees

required for the degree because of time constraints. The degree did not seem necessary to me at the time because I already had a master's degree, though 16 years later I see that it might serve as a credentialling positive against future events.

These courses spanned several years and provided much of the formal preparation for my long-time goal. When I began as Director of Social Work at Harborview, I discussed my career goals with the administrator who promptly expanded my responsibilities to include other departments. By 1970, I was on my way, intrigued by the new challenges and providing new leadership and direction within the administrative circle of the hospital. Thus, while I was motivated to absorb new administrative challenges, the administrator was also eager for me to assume responsibility for some "trouble-spots" and areas which required an infusion of leadership and morale building. The combination worked well and by 1980 I had acquired incrementally several increased responsibilities culminating in my appointment in 1981 as assistant administrator. My workload also increased proportionally to the new responsibilities necessitating my working well over the traditional 40 hour week. Juggling both the administrator role and the academic roles has been difficult at times. Both require enormous amounts of time, specifically during the hospital budgeting cycle and the academic quarters in which I teach. In addition, the specialty field of family and interpersonal violence has literally exploded over the past dozen years creating not only opportunities for systems innovations and clinical practice, but also a tremendous demand for coursework and additional education for all health care professionals. The challenge for me has been to combine efforts among competing roles, that of administrator, academician, clinical expert and social work director. That challenge continues to serve me well and provide impetus for developing new programs, new legislation, new clinical efforts including grant writing as well as creating an atmosphere in which others under my supervision and direction can contribute effectively. I have been continually impressed with the abilities of those for whom I am responsible as they carve out their own specialty areas, advance programs, write major articles for publication and provide leadership to others. Modeling has been, for me, a rewarding experience. I think it works well in producing future leaders in the health care system.

Time has been one of the most critical areas to manage and the one which has been the most difficult. While the social work staff was pleased and proud of my new administrative responsibilities, they soon came to learn its cost in my having less available time. But this was not necessarily negative. This dilemma created the opportunities for new managers and new leadership within the Social Work Department through empowerment and delegation of authority. In all ways, this has strengthened the department and added to its overall visibility in the hospital and community.

Being a social worker in a hospital administration has not always been as rewarding or positive as one might expect. There have been many myths to overcome. For instance, social work does not have a strong image as hospital administrator or fiscal manager. Many physicians see social work as a "soft" or unstructured discipline. On the other hand, there are also myths that stereotype administrators as tough, fiscal disciplinarians or the contrary, as weak and unable to make decisions. What counts in the final analysis is the outcome, the process by which that occurs and the steps in the process. I brought a particular sense of process to management, of fairness and equity, of empowerment, of "win-wins" and options for problem solutions. These attributes are part of social work ethics and values to which we continually dedicate ourselves. They work well for me as a social work director and hospital administrator.

MANAGEMENT SKILLS

Charles Garfield (1984), believes that peak-performing leaders are trained, not born. He details ten qualities of high performing managers which contribute significantly to their success. These qualities merit review and discussion to identify what contributes to effective leadership and management and how it can be taught. Although the qualities here refer to managers in the generic sense, by implication they apply to social work administrators and leaders. Garfield notes that peak performing managers:

1. exhibit foresight and the ability to execute effective strategic planning. The focus is on long-term planning and goals and away from a short-sighted approach.
2. decide in advance what staffing, equipment, finances and other resources they will need to successfully complete a project.
3. refuse to become entrapped at any particular plateau for very long. The aim is away from the status quo and consistently toward higher levels of accomplishment through excellence and attainment of specific goals.
4. possess a superior ability to take creative risks thus avoiding prolonged "comfort zones."
5. demonstrate high levels of self-confidence and self-worth.
6. have a significant need for responsibility and control. They are not afraid to take action and seldom feel victimized.
7. mentally rehearse key situations by envisioning both the process and the desired outcome.
8. tend to engage in their work for the art and passion of it. They approach their "mission" with enthusiasm.

9. concentrate on problem-solving rather than placing blame. They avoid behaviors which are self-defeating and counterproductive.
10. demonstrate a proprietary attitude—that is, they have a tendency to assume ownership of their ideas and products.

These ten "qualities" were certainly guides for me and can be guides for social workers who aspire to supervisory as well as administrative positions. They easily lend themselves to a curriculum in which they can be taught, and as such are not exclusive to one discipline but offer attainable goals for all types of administrators.

Social Work brings a unique contribution to the management forum which provides further implications for graduate school curricula. My academic preparation in group work, community organization and public administration became the foundation for movement into hospital administration. Further, preparation in finding and establishing environmental resources and bringing them to the [administrative] experience is unique, historically, to the social work profession. We are experts at understanding environmental effects on individuals and their families. This factor alone contributes to strategic long term planning and the foresight required by the health care system. Secondly, the "systems-approach" to problem solving, which was a major emphasis in my social work education, contributed significantly to comfort with absorbing administrative responsibilities and the administrative role. Thirdly, the ecological perspective of the bio-psycho-social approach emphasizes a social work mission and function(s) which involve community organization and social planning, both necessary ingredients in today's health care world.

An avid feminist in the holistic sense, I also brought a feminist perspective, addressing the issues of empowerment, equity and fairness, egalitarian commitment and assertiveness in the administrative role. While these are articulated social work values, it has only been with the advent of the women's movement that these specific qualities, skills, indeed knowledge base, have taken on new meaning through new translations. The same skills applicable in quality clinical social work are easily integrated into health care administration. Settings may differ and situations may call for different orders of knowledge and different sets of criteria with which to evaluate success, but many of the basic elements inherent in the social work profession fit this new and emerging managerial role.

I found that other qualities, knowledge and skills are additionally requisite to effective administration. A manager or administrator is also an organizational planner, a leader, an organizer, a controller. In fact, management per se is often referred to as the "process of planning, organizing, leading, and controlling the efforts of organizational members and the use of organizational resources in order to achieve stated organizational goals" (Stoner, 1978[A], p. 7). Social work administrators perform all these tasks but possess essential academic preparation and oftentimes job training which enhance their administrative abilities. Social work preparation combined with the qualities, traits and characteristics of leadership produces dynamic and avant-garde administrators in today's health care industry. Social work's social mission and dedication to helping people directly or through systems, its philosophical stance of the person-in-situation, its ability to connect people with resources in their environment and the inherent processes which enable the formation of these connections, provide a distinct and exceptional preparation for administrative leadership in the social health care delivery system. Further, the successful administrator is a conceptual as well as an analytical thinker who first approaches the entire task in the abstract, conceptualizing the organizational planning aspect in the broader context, while at the same time analyzing the needed step-by-step implementation strategies. Both are requisite to an effective and holistic administrative knowledge and skill base. Additionally, a creative and effective administrator works with and through other people to achieve the desired organizational goals. In this context the administrator becomes a conduit of information and acts as a channel of communication. Thus, social work's skills in the understanding and management of "process" becomes a valuable and distinctive knowledge and skill base. Social work administrators are well prepared for another managerial role, that of mediator. Social work preparation in methods, themes, assumptions and values specific to the social and psychological components in human behavior are applicable and germane to the alleviation and resolution of most administrative problem solving tasks.

The administrator also makes politic use of compromise, persuasion, coercion, bargaining, collaborating and other means to promote organizational effectiveness. In this context, the administrator is a diplomat, balancing competing and often conflicting goals and objectives. Again, social work preparation and training specifically address, through the profession's ethical and value stance, the art of compromise, of listening to and exploring all sides of issues and evaluating all information. The process by which this occurs is inherent in social work education and practice.

Managers from all arenas take on a wide range of tasks, activities and roles. By focusing on what effective managers do, we can explicate what an effective manager is. The following roles and activities are characteristic, major managerial undertakings. Effective managers for the most part are able to:

1. assume responsibility and insure that tasks are completed successfully;
2. balance many competing goals;

3. translate their vision, insight and imagination into action planning;
4. organize by creative coordination the human and material resources of the organization;
5. strategically negotiate differences and conflicts;
6. collaborate with and influence others;
7. advocate and broker for services, programs and resources;
8. innovate, create and develop programs;
9. implement goals through enabling structures;
10. influence in the political sense using timing as a necessary creative skill;
11. evaluate outcomes and adopt changes through dynamic processes;
12. prepare and empower others to create a dynamic and strengthened program/unit/department.

Social work administrators perform these activities and roles based on their commitment to the bio-psycho-social aspects of illness and wellness within the concept of continuity of care. This clinical perspective is essential in today's health care system and offers the health care industry a unique complement to existing managerial roles. What emerges is a more comprehensive and dynamic administrative leadership style. Indeed at this time health care systems need humanistic as well as efficient managers and it is logical that social workers increasingly are tapped to fill managerial positions in health care settings. The broader leadership role itself requires a detailed scrutiny and elaboration.

LEADERSHIP

Leadership ability is one of the more if not the most important qualities in establishing the successful and effective administrator. One can have imagination, knowledge, skills and preparation, but leadership ability is the "cement" that integrates them. Skillful leadership creates the processes of the effective and successful manager.

In spite of many studies of leaders and their characteristics, exact knowledge in this area is limited. We often speak of the natural traits such as "star qualities," charisma, intensity, persuasiveness, and foresight which emerge as reasonably common characteristics among well-known historical figures. The key to understanding leadership and leadership style is to "learn the behaviors and techniques, thereby improving our personal and organizational effectiveness" (Stoner, 1978[B], p. 437). Further, if we can isolate and identify these qualities we can better prepare social workers to become administrators not only in health care but in a variety of other settings as well.

There are almost as many definitions of leadership as there are studies.

For purposes of this discussion, leadership is defined as the process of directing and influencing activities of group members. It is based on three important assumptions. One, leadership must involve other people, subordinates and superiors. Two, the leadership process involves unequal distribution of power. There must be a hierarchical distribution of power particularly in a bureaucratic structure. That is, some have more decision-making authority or power than others. Three, leaders can influence subordinates and others in the hierarchy in addition to providing direction to them (Stoner, 1978[B], p. 438).

Effective leadership in health care today takes place in a climate of constant changes in our social and health care systems. An effective health care leader will anticipate these changes and respond to the critical trends in our health care system, as, for example, cost containment and cost reduction efforts by government and the private sector; new financing systems for hospitals emphasizing ambulatory care models and cost sharing by consumers; experimentation with alternative health delivery systems; development of primary and preventive health services; emphasis on post-hospital and after-care services; increased emphasis on services to the aging and elderly; continued explosion of high technological advances; increasing issues of availability, access, continuity and quality of care; growth of complex value and ethical dilemmas with debates over priorities and use of scarce resources; continued emphasis on the interface between social, legal and health systems such as in issues of family and other manifestations of interpersonal violence. These are but some of the more pressing societal trends which affect leaders in the health care system and especially challenge the social work profession to prepare and respond to new opportunities in managerial leadership.

An important component of the nature of leadership is power or empowerment and any discussion of leadership requires some discussion of power. As with leadership, much has been written and studied about power and power sources. Most notable is the work of French and Raven (1959) who delineate five essential bases of power.

1. *Reward Power*: the power to reward or compensate another for tasks successfully completed.
2. *Coercive Power*: the ability to punish for not carrying out tasks.
3. *Legitimate Power*: formal authority or power of lawful influence.
4. *Referent Power*: the power to cause others to identify with or imitate (the leader's) behavior, style.
5. *Expert Power*: the power of superior knowledge, ability or skill.

Obviously, the more sources of power and influence a leader possesses, the more effective the leadership. In fact, some scholars imply that the number of power bases alone may separate mediocre from superior leaders and administrators.

Planning is the first step in building power bases. But even prior to the initiation of tasks, one must be comfortable with power and empowerment, i.e., wearing power (self-esteem and modeling) and giving power (delegation and empowerment). Power or social power as discussed by Wax (1968), has come to have a negative connotation for some and sometimes is confused with politics, another word with negative overtones. Both power and politics are definite realities of the business world of which health care is an integral part. Social work has much to learn from business but we must first feel comfortable with the issues of power. We must give ourselves permission to succeed, to win, and to achieve, to take and give power. Social workers can be change agents in health care settings.

Stoner (1978[B], p. 439) further elaborates our understanding of leadership by discussing three major approaches to the study of leadership. The first and least productive approach is based on the search for leadership traits. These studies fail to identify specific traits which are useful in denoting or predicting leadership abilities (Vroom, 1978). Attempting to profile leadership this way seems akin to attempts at profiling the characteristics of alcoholics or sexual offenders. Identifiable characteristics or traits apply to non-leaders as well as leaders, to non-alcoholics as well as alcoholics and to non-offenders as well as sexual offenders. "Most studies in this area have found that effective leadership did not depend on a particular set of traits but on how well the leader's traits matched the requirements of the situation (Cartwright and Zander, 1968). Again, the process stands out as the key element.

A second approach tries to identify the essence of leadership by examining behaviors that make leaders effective. Researchers tried to determine what effective leaders do, i.e., how they delegate, how they communicate, how they motivate. These studies are based on the assumption that behaviors are learned and can be taught. This approach, however, resulted in identification of many non-transferable behaviors; that behaviors appropriate in one situation were not necessarily appropriate to another. Nevertheless, these studies have proved useful and effective in their focus on leadership functions and leadership styles, the most effective of which seems to emerge as a flexible style.

Emanating from the first two, a third approach focuses on situational and environmental factors in effective leadership, factors such as organizational climate, policies, managerial values, and experience. The point is that no one leadership trait or style was most effective in all situations (Dannette, 1976). Instead, identifying the total aspect of the situation including the leader's personality, past experiences, the superior's expectations and·behavior, the subordinate's characteristics, expectations and behavior, the requirements of the tasks to be performed, and peer expectation and behavior, are all contributory to effective leadership (Stoner, 1978[B], p. 448).

Finally, the three approaches mentioned give way to various contingency approaches to leadership (Stoner, 1978[B], p. 452). These approaches, probably more reflective of social work theory and practice, attempt to identify which of these factors is more important in a given situation and to predict the leadership style that will be most effective in that situation, again emphasizing the essential need for flexibility. Of many models available, one in particular, Hershey and Blanchard's life cycle theory of leadership (Stoner, 1978[B], p. 458), suggests that leadership style varies with the maturity of subordinates and with the specifics of situations. Maturity refers to desire for achievement, willingness to accept responsibilities and tasks, related ability and experience. The manager-subordinate relationship moves through different phases as subordinates develop achievement, motivation, and experience (Stoner, 1978[B], p. 461). Here again, emphasis is on flexibility based on the specific situation. The surviving organization is the adaptive one. The surviving leader is the adaptive and flexible leader. The leader, in touch with all the "pieces" and "players," the inside and outside world, senses change and adapts to it. Peters and Austin (1985) illustrate that flexible leadership *is* the difference between success or failure. They note from their study that successful leaders provided latitude but were tough taskmasters who challenged, demanded, and rewarded excellence.

Much like the social work steps of study, diagnosis and treatment, the manager-leader can learn to diagnose a situation, can utilize a variety of styles and effect appropriate leadership as the major goal in administering. What is important is that along with specific and identifiable qualities, tasks and responsibilities which spell "success," leadership provides the structures, mechanisms and processes through which effective and quality administration can occur. Leadership capability becomes the nuts and bolts of the organization. Many researchers have indicated that the critical element in an organization's overall success is the ability to select managers with high leadership capabilities.

CONCLUSION

The state of today's health care system has critical importance for the professional social worker in administration. Issues related to health status, health care organization, health care policy, and health care accessibility are pressing challenges in which social workers can make dynamic contributions as leaders.

It is clear in reviewing the early historical roots of the social work profession that these contributions are congruent with the social health issues current in our nation. Our heritage is in working with the poor, the disadvantaged, the homeless, in helping people better themselves within the values and ethics of self-determination. The sense of mastery, autonomy, empowerment and competency for positive change are outcomes for which we aim, whether in clinical or administrative practice. Skills in achieving these outcomes are applicable and transferable to health care administration.

The nature and scope of comtemporary health problems demand a bio-psycho-social approach and social work provides this important comprehensive view. Specifically, medical conditions such as hypertension and cardiovascular disease, cancer, stroke, diabetes, alcoholism, substance abuse, mental illness, end-stage renal disease, problems of the elderly, sexually transmitted diseases, accidents, suicides, environmental hazards, and interpersonal violence are but some examples which demand a bio-psycho-social perspective. Particularly important is our profession's approach to ethical dilemmas, to quality of life issues, and to its major emphasis on prevention.

Entering health care administration from social work has been challenging and rewarding for me. The knowledge, skills, values and techniques inherent in the social work profession can enhance the administrator's role and effectiveness. These qualities, discussed earlier, include (1) the social-systems environment, (2) the bio-psycho-social or ecological perspective, and (3) the person-in-situation or environment context.

In Ann Hartman's (1980) discussion of the clinical competencies of social work which are transferable to administrative practice, she notes special competencies unique to social work. We bring a holistic, person-in-situation, life space approach to assessment, an "exploratory" stance which especially prepares the social work administrator to competently and courageously explore all variables in a management situation. Social work brings a systems perspective which calls for a multi-dimensional examination and ordering of data in the analytic and integrative phases of planning. Social work offers special interpersonal skills in identifying, reaching out and engaging special populations to be served, skills which are pertinent and indispensible in the complex relationships with the multiple constituencies with whom an administrator deals. As administrators we can use our social work principle of self-determination; we can make connections and bridge social distances in planning and implementing programs in our health care delivery systems. Our social work skills in negotiating, in engaging client participation and in contracting can be applied to all levels of planning and engagement. Egalitarianism, realism, open communication and empowerment are tools similarly useful in the processes of management.

In summary, there is much in specific knowledge and skills that social work can bring to the arena of health care administration. A task which we must assume is that of educating other disciplines in the health care setting regarding social work's contributions. I was able through actual clinical practice in my early years to demonstrate the effectiveness and importance of psycho-social assessment and diagnosis and its usefulness in medical compliance. The development of clinical protocols, for which the Harborview Social Work Department is well known, has served to standardize the role and functions of social work, thereby educating the health care team. By demonstrating what social workers do by task and responsibility, and connecting these to outcome(s), we demonstrate to other professionals our value and effect on the health care delivery system. Social work is taking the lead today in developing ethics committees and ethic forums in hospitals. Social work is having an impact on effective and appropriate discharge planning and length of stay under the current cost reimbursement system. Social work activities with community systems, in enacting legislation and in assisting with issues of access to health care which extend services to many vulnerable populations, are a few examples of our influence in the management arena. Social work's contributions to management can be significant; they illustrate how social work as the profession of choice can advance the role of the successful manager/administrator in the social health care of our nation.

REFERENCES

Cartwright, Darwin, & Zander, Alvin (Eds.). *Group Dynamics*, 3rd ed. New York: Harper and Row, 1968.

Dannette, D. (Ed.). *Handbook of Industrial and Organizational Psychology*. Chicago: Rand McNally, 1976.

Garfield, Charles A. *Peak Performance*. Tarcher/Houghton Miffin, 1984.

Hartman, Ann. "Competencies in Clinical Social Work." *Toward a Definition of Clinical Social Work*. NASW Conference Proceedings, January 1980.

French, John R. O. & Raven, Bertram. "The Bases of Social Power." In Darwin Cartwright (Ed.), *Studies in Social Power*. University of Michigan, 1959, pp. 150–167.

Peters, Tom & Austin, Nancy. *A Passion for Excellence, the Leadership Difference*. Random House, Inc., 1985.

Stoner, James. "Managing and Managers." *Management*. New Jersey: Prentice-Hall, 1978(A).

Stoner, James. "Leadership." *Management*. New Jersey: Prentice-Hall, 1978(B).

Vroom, Victor. "Leadership." *Management*. New Jersey: Prentice-Hall, 1978, pp. 440, 441.

Wax, John. "Developing Social Work Power in a Medical Organization." *Social Work*. 1968.

CHAPTER VI

Social Work and Hospital Administration

Harold L. Light, MSS

MY TRANSITION

After five years of pre-Master's degree employment as a case worker in the New York City Bureau of Child Welfare (three years in child placement and two years in the supervision of foster homes) and almost three years of post-Master's degree employment as a family counselor and group therapist in a family service agency, I was employed as the Director of Social Work Services for a free standing ambulatory care center affiliated with the Beth Israel Medical Center in New York City. The ambulatory care center was to become a prototypical "family care center" which ultimately served as a model for the Office of Economic Opportunity's nationwide program for neighborhood health care centers. New York City, similarly, patterned its neighborhood family care center program after the ambulatory care unit.

Because the ambulatory care unit was located on the lower east side of Manhattan where five well-established settlement houses had developed through the periods of great in-migration; because a number of other social agencies and community organizations had developed through the years to service the various social, emotional and economic needs of the population; and because the health care unit was established with its most basic philosophical premise being that it would be an entity "of the community" rather than "for the community," there was a purposeful and natural evolution of an organizational structure which placed the Director of Social Work Services into a pivotal position within the organizational hierarchy (Light and Brown, 1964).

Included in the earliest of responsibilities assumed by me within the organization were overall responsibility for the human resources function and a community organization function along the lines more character- istically reserved for professional community organizers. The human resources functions included responsibility for *all* personnel in the organization including members of the Medical Staff. (It is noteworthy that all of the physicians providing care at the unit were salaried and none was a "voluntary staff" physician within the organization though many held voluntary Medical Staff appointments at Beth Israel Medical Center and at other voluntary teaching hospitals in New York City.) Literally, every employee hired by the organization was interviewed by me with an eye toward determining that individual's ability to grasp the nature of the unit's mission and with an eye toward screening out individuals at any level who had difficulty accepting the basic underlying precepts of the organization.

The quick and eager acceptance by the community's social work power structure of my role as principal communicator, liaison person and ex- pediter of services for their clients helped to solidify my position as a member of the "Administration." Three months after my arrival as Di- rector of Social Work Services, I was given the additional title of Assistant Administrator and served in both capacities for nine months while the Administrator, a more traditionally trained graduate of the Columbia School of Public Health, went about organizing the business and account- ing functions, developing the purchasing and receiving functions, creating an environmental atmosphere intended to make the facility an attractive place to visit and dealing with other aspects of the administrative function generally reserved for traditional "line administrators" within health care organizations.

Nine months after my having been given responsibilities as the Assistant Administrator, the Administrator left the organization to assume another position. At that time, the Medical Director of the unit and his adminis- trative superiors at the Beth Israel Medical Center were faced with making a determination about the individual who would become successor to the Administrator. After a fairly extensive search and many interviews with experienced hospital administrators, almost all of whom were graduates of Master's degree programs in Public Health, Hospital Administration or Business Administration, a determination was made that the needs of the organization would be better served by an individual whose social phi- losophy paralleled the already established philosophy of the health care unit and who could learn the rudiments of the "business aspects" required by the position rather than engaging an individual already educated in the business areas and infusing him or her with a philosophy that paralleled that of the organization. Once that determination had been made, the search process stopped and the position was offered to me. Once again, this position was assumed without surrendering the directorship of Social

Work Services and with no dimunition in responsibilities for the human resources function. This dual responsibility continued for an additional two and one-half years at which time, because of an ongoing assumption of additional activities and responsibilities, a Director of Social Work Services was hired with a direct reporting relationship to me.

Two years later, when the unit was well established and serving as a model for other such units and when a new facility to house the services had been planned and designed, I resigned my position to assume the position of Special Assistant for Ambulatory Care Planning within the newly created municipal "super agency" called the Health Systems Agency. One year later, having completed work in helping to design the neighborhood family care center program for New York City, I left to take my first position within another hospital where, once again, my primary responsibilities were for Ambulatory Care Services, the Social Work function, the Home Care function and all activities involving community programs. Following that experience, I became Deputy Director of Long Island Jewish/Hillside Medical Center where the Social Work function reported to me for the first several years of my tenure. After seven years of experience at that institution, I assumed the position of President and Chief Executive Officer of The Long Island College Hospital in Brooklyn, New York where the nature and scope of responsibilities of my position preclude the possibility of any direct supervisory relationship with the Social Work function.

In the career progression described above, I never reached out for additional or changed responsibilities. Most of the career moves made, however, were made during a period of rapid growth of the health care industry following the passage of Medicare and Medicaid legislation when hospital expansion resulted in administrative openings and when hospital executives and Boards were seeking energetic individuals who accepted the notion that health care was a right rather than a privilege and that the health care system was part of the country's social fabric and deserved to be treated as such.

In large measure, each of the career moves I made was rationalized as a natural progression toward positions of greater responsibility and influence which could, by the very nature of their position in the respective organizational hierarchies in which I found myself, lead to a greater humanization of the health care delivery system.

UTILITY AND LIMITS OF SOCIAL WORK FOR HOSPITAL MANAGEMENT

In assessing the factors which made it possible for a Master's degree social worker to move into a position of authority in health care administration, I put aside factors relating to intelligence, education and special knowledge because, as I see it, virtually every Master's degree social worker in the country has the intellectual capacity to acquire knowledge if he or she wanted to take the time and trouble to read the myriad journals and publications produced within the field and, certainly, each has the capacity to absorb the contents of an academic program in health care administration if one had the time and economic wherewithal to interrupt a career for the purpose of acquiring such an education. Such people, however, were they starting on such a career path today, would be disadvantaged by the absence of some of the "on the job training" opportunities afforded those who entered the field during its time of expansion and would be disadvantaged, as well, by the assaults being made on the health care industry for that very same growth and for what has been called an "unbridled" increase in expenditures in the health care field.

Nevertheless, behaviorists, in increasing numbers, are assuming positions of administrative responsibility in health care settings and it is understandable that they should do so. Debates about the appropriate percentage of the gross national product which should be spent on health care notwithstanding, there is little doubt that most social workers view health care as an entitlement similar to that of public education. Similarly, there is little doubt that behaviorists are opposed to the rationing of health care, believe in the right of self-determination relative to health care needs, (including such controversial issues as abortion and the right to die with dignity), believe in active and informed participation in the decision making process relating to ones health care needs, believe in the access to all levels of sophisticated care irrespective of race, color, creed, ethnicity, national origin or sexual preference, believe that advocacy on behalf of the patient is an appropriate role and function for themselves and support the notion that sensitivity to the patients' psychological and emotional needs are equal in importance to physical considerations.

One cannot ignore the fact that there are personality and "natural" qualities of leadership without which no individual, irrespective of his or her level of intellect and irrespective of his or her acquired knowledge about the health care field could succeed as an administrator (Peters and Waterman, 1982). We are all familiar with the charismatic individual who is able to lead large numbers of people and to affect the shape and nature of an organization despite the fact that he or she may know little about that organization's internal operations.

On the other hand, the extraordinarily complex nature of hospital administration, particularly of the teaching hospital which is Medical School affiliated, makes it impossible in today's climate for any administrator to be successful on the basis of personality or charisma alone.

Some have suggested that the administrator who does not control the means of production (the voluntary staff physician who admits patients to the hospital and thereby generates most of its income) and who is powerless to establish the price for his organization's services, (reimbursement rates are set by others) is doomed to failure. When one compounds those liabilities with the pressures which are brought to bear by members of the Board of Trustees who frequently are themselves managers of organizations which are not so constrained, it is easy to understand why the "life expectancy" of the hospital administrator in his role as manager is as short lived as it has turned out to be.

Behaviorists in general, and social workers in particular, do develop, by virtue of their education and training, various skills, qualities and characteristics which can be helpful in a successful career in administration if many of the knowledge factors and personality traits previously referred to are also in place. For example, there is probably no organizational structure where the ability to understand latent communication is as important as it is in a teaching hospital; there is probably no organizaiton which is populated by more "rugged individualists" (physicians) whose very education and training are such as to make them individual decision makers as opposed to those who subordinate their own needs to a group process. Surely, the ability to listen with "a third ear" and the ability to bring groups of people to a common understanding through a group process are skills acquired by most social workers through the years. When one combines those abilities with the ability to conceptualize philosophies and goals and with one's ability to recognize and work within a highly politicized organizational framework, the likelihood of being able to advance one's self in the administrative hierarchy is strengthened.

At one and the same time, many of those same characteristics and qualities are factors which can ensure one's inability to advance administratively. Social workers in hospitals are, by definition, intruders in a host agency which sees itself as being, principally, a workshop of the medical practitioner. By definition these individuals believe they should make policy for the institution, that the institution is there to serve their needs and that the operation of the institution should be so organized as to be convenient to their office hour schedules. Those who represent a strenuous advocacy position for the patient or who represent a philosophic position which suggests that patient care institutions should focus first and foremost on the needs of the patient are likely to find themselves at odds with the medical power structure. When such individuals also believe they have a responsibility to identify deficits in the quality of medical care being provided, they are likely to find themselves in a constant state of war with a powerful and potentially vengeful force.

IMPLICATIONS

Can social workers, or anyone for that matter, be prepared for a successful career in hospital administration through a formal educational process? Are the generic elements of administration such as to suggest that many of the post Master's degree curricula being offered by schools of social work are as applicable to the health care field as they are to the field of social work administration? Can any school adequately screen candidates for administrative sequences so as to ensure that those who emerge from the didactic process will be able to carry what they have learned into a real life situation?

My own sense is that it would be wasteful and unproductive for schools of social work to create a health care administrative sequence. As the operation of hospitals becomes more business-like, as the number of acute care beds continues to shrink and as the number of acute care hospitals continues to decline via closings resulting from under-utilization, existing schools of business and hospital administration are likely to be producing more graduates than there are jobs. Some of these declines will be offset by the expansion of long term care facilities which will also require sophisticated management, but the likelihood is that we will continue to see a surplus of graduates for the foreseeable future (Starr, 1982).

None of this is intended to suggest, however, that social workers with the qualities, traits and interests described earlier cannot strive for administrative positions in health care facilities. The realities of life do suggest that such candidates will be disadvantaged in a competitive environment and will have to be extraordinarily fortunate to be given the opportunity to prove their abilities.

REFERENCES

Light, Harold L. and Brown, Howard J. "The Social Worker as Lay Administrator of a Medical Facility," *Social Casework*, June 1964.
Peters, Thomas J. and Waterman, Robert H. *In Search of Excellence*. Harper and Row, New York, 1982.
Starr, Paul. *The Social Transformation of American Medicine*, New York: Basic Books, 1982.

CHAPTER VII

Administration:
Getting the Right Things Done

Stanley K. Nielson, ACSW

CURRENT POSITION AND RESPONSIBILITIES

I am the Executive Director of a not-for-profit corporation named *Commonhealth, Inc.* It is a service component of a larger health care corporation called General Health Services, Inc. This larger corporation evolved as a result of a complex series of reorganization moves originating in an acute care hospital, Madison General Hospital. This reorganization was influenced by political and governmental pressures as well as internal hospital actions which sought to cope with the economic and financial stresses of cost containment, declining census, diversification of health delivery, and a very fluid environment which made Madison, Wisconsin the hotbed of national HMO development. General Health Services, Inc., is the corporate parent for a series of other corporations which represent for-profit and not-for-profit entities.

Commonhealth, Inc., although only two years old as of this writing, occupies a unique presence in our community in that it represents a merger of city government interests and a health corporation's desires to focus on the community health care needs of its vulnerable citizens. Commonhealth has established several main efforts.

1. It will work jointly with all existing agencies in ensuring that identified health care needs of vulnerable populations are being met;
2. It will serve as a major advocacy agency within the governmental public policy arena and within the general business environment to ensure that the population's health care needs are being dealt with;
3. Commonhealth will work with agencies in developing projects and

---

The author is now Director, Patient and Family Services, Meritor/Madison General Hospital, Madison, WI.

programs that enable citizens to better access the health and welfare systems;

4. It will take leadership in developing services to meet health care needs of citizens and provide those services when it appears no existing agency or entity will currently assume that responsibility. These services will be developed with short term objectives and with the major thrust of enabling existing agencies to eventually assume these responsibilities;

5. Commonhealth also will assume a major role in educating the general public, its clients, and its resource system about health and health related issues which may impact the community.

In the local jargon of our community, Commonhealth, Inc., "helps others to help others."

My major role in Commonhealth, as Executive Director, is to work with my Board of Directors in developing the agency's goals and objectives, ensuring the mechanisms for their attainment, and creating the necessary support systems to assist the agency in its activities. This entails budget development and fiscal supports, creation of management information systems, manpower resource development, and evaluating the overall performance of the organization. Along with this is a significant expectation of personal involvement in behind the scenes political advocacy and lobbying with all levels of the health and welfare scene and where necessary, overtly with the political system of government itself at any level appropriate to the attainment of agency goals.

I occupy a rather unique position as Executive Director of Commonhealth because I am a corporate employee of a management company owned by the corporate parent. I am not appointed to my lead position by my agency Board yet I am fully accountable for what my Board does, says, develops, and directs me to fulfill. It is a position known as "being between a rock and a hard place." I deal with health and welfare issues on a daily basis yet do not operate as part of our established health and welfare system in our community. My current Board has eleven members, six chosen by the Corporate office from the community and five chosen by the mayor of our community. These five currently represent a cross-section of low income and special interest group advocates for expanded health care services. This combination of people, all very dedicated to Commonhealth's growth and influence potential in the community, creates an exciting challenge for the director.

THE TRANSITION

My involvement in Commonhealth arose partially from career transition and from the organizational redesign of my previous employer,

Madison General Hospital. I had been employed by the hospital for 15 years; first as the Director of the Patient Services Department for 10 years and then as Assistant Vice-President for Diagnostic and Treatment Services. Initially responsible for the leadership and development of the social services and home care (discharge planning) system of the hospital, I was moved into the administrative echelon where I was responsible for the administrative organization, direction, implementation, control, and evaluation of the acute care hospital's physical medicine, psychiatric and substance abuse programs. I therefore moved through the ensuing years from a department head carrying an active social work role and a managerial role, to purely a managerial role within a social work department, and then to an administrative position which was purely managerial in nature.

Over the past several years, the acute care hospital encountered the same economic and political pressures experienced across the nation. We encountered job actions, declining patient census, consolidations of nursing units, numerous changes in our managerial structures, and an ever-pressuring fiscal posture of prudent resource allocation and a finely tuned delivery system. As a responsible manager and administrator, I participated actively in the redefinition of our facility's mission, its resultant changes in its delivery capability, and the modifications necessary to cope with declining resources. It was very evident that restructuring the program elements responsible to me was a necessary direction in keeping with administrative goals and objectives. Over an eight month period, I worked with my administrative colleagues in streamlining our managerial system at all levels, including top administration. Even as the Vice-President with the major seniority, prudent administrative redesign indicated that my position was no longer necessary. Creating one's own demise was a major challenge and I will acknowledge that despite its intrigue and the learning experience it provided, certain anxieties and trepidations occurred. The administrative support was present as the process ensued, particularly from the top executive, but my peer administrative colleagues were so anxious that they provided little to no support for me.

Although offered another administrative position in the hospital, my assessment of this position and redefinition of my own professional skills and goals indicated that at best the proffered position was a holding pattern for me. I was also becoming distressed over the rapidly evolving "bottom line" mentality and the sacrifice of some strong institutional social values and community responsiveness.

As the hospital was reorganizing, the overall corporate structure was also developing. Responding to community pressures, the corporation was having to redefine what its corporate mission in community service was to be and through what medium it would carry out that role. A community services corporation was developed and although its mission was very ambiguous, it nevertheless met the community's desires. I was initially asked to be a member of the organization's Board and assist the parent corporation to administratively structure it, attain its not-for-profit status, and begin working within the Board to more concretely develop its mission, goals and objectives, budget, and internal structure. The existing potential of this new corporate entity, its unique position in a corporate system that could possibly influence public policy, and its even more intriguing position in the community, stimulated my interests so much that I actively sought the Executive Director post being developed. I received substantial encouragement from many people within and outside the corporation. I entered the competition for the position and was eventually appointed Executive Director.

SOCIAL WORK AND MANAGEMENT SKILL

As I look back upon my professional career as a social work clinician, as a social work manager, as an administrator within a health care system, and now as a chief executive officer of a corporation, I am struck by the impact of some of the social work framework provided me through formal education and pure experience.

Although brought up in the old social work era of casework, group work, and community organization, I find all three practice arenas particularly important in my current position. The focus or "client" is ever-changing. In the mid-seventies, Pincus and Minahan (1973) of the University of Wisconsin School of Social Work developed a practice model which provided a base for a generalist practitioner as opposed to the specialist. It set a foundation for either one, depending on how the practitioner built upon it and incorporated his/her special knowledge and interests regarding particular social problems, client groups, resource systems, theoretical orientations, and social science knowledge.

A quote that remains in my mind and with a few word substitutions could apply to a social work manager, an administrator or chief executive officer read as follows:

> Social work is concerned with the interactions between people and their social environment which affect the ability of people to accomplish their life tasks, alleviate distress, and realize their aspirations and values. The purpose of social work therefore is to (1) enhance the problem-solving and coping capacities of people, (2) link people with systems that provide them with resources, services, and opportunities, (3) promote the effective and humane operation of these systems, and (4) contribute to the development and improvement of social policy.

It is obvious to me from experience that regardless of our role, we function as change agents and are always engaged in planned change efforts. We need to decide what our purposes and relationships should be in working through the change process. We need to be clear who will benefit from our change efforts, who will need to be changed or influenced, and whom we will need to work with in order to achieve different goals in our change efforts. These activities can be viewed in relation to four types of systems: change agent, client, target, and action. These can be defined as:

1. *Change agent:* The change agent and the people who are part of his employing organization.
2. *Client system:* People who sanction or ask for the change agent's services, who are the expected beneficiaries of service, and who have a working agreement or contract with the change agent.
3. *Target system:* People who need to be changed to accomplish the goals of the change agent.
4. *Action system:* The change agent and the people he works with and through to accomplish his goals and influence the target system.

Any social worker contemplating advancement into management and higher administration must be aware of the complexity of their own organization or other organization offering that advancement. They better be! Health care organizations are complex institutions that require ever-higher levels of sophistication on the part of those who manage them. Sophisticated managers make decisions using cognitive skills that combine a substantial knowledge base with the ability to analyze and synthesize data, in order to identify problems and to develop strategies and options for their resolution.

Being a good manager requires more than having a kit of "how to" skills. It is unproductive to give managers techniques for making decisions, planning, organizing, executing or controlling without providing clues about what needs to be decided and planned and to what end to organize, execute, and control. Such techniques constitute an important part of the skill base managers must acquire. These cognitive skills are not dissimilar to those of a good social work clinician, whose understanding of the client and the multitude of influences shaping that client is the base for clinical decisions.

The practice of management also demands a range of perspectives. Perspectives limited to the psychology of individuals and groups (micro) or to the sociology of organizations (macro) can skew one's vision and misdirect managerial work. To be effective, managers must balance their concerns about people in the organization with the needs of the organization as a whole. Knowledge in both areas, and the ability to apply it to the mutual advantage of people and of the organization as a whole, is a cognitive skill all too infrequently addressed.

These ideas about cognitive skills of effective managers can be refined into two interrelated parts, each having a general knowledge base and a specific application. The first is a knowledge about organizations, and the second is knowledge about the work of management.

Charns and Schaefer (1983) provide a wealth of information on the organizational environment. Their basic thrust is to assist the manager in understanding organizations and how they work and to learn how to work within them. They recognize that organizations and open systems exist in and interact with their environments, that organizations exist to do work, and that the requirements for organizations depend upon the characteristics of work. There is obviously a definite focus on *work* in the organizational model but explicit attention is given to management work as being different from direct work. The work of managing a health services organization is different from the work of providing care to a patient, even though they are interrelated and sometimes provided by the same person. Thus there are two task systems, one for the direct work of the organization and another for the management work.

After a review of the literature it is obvious that there are almost as many definitions of management as there are writers in the field. A common trend appearing in these definitions is the managers concern for accomplishing organizational goals and objectives. Hersey and Blanchard (1982) boil down all these definitions into a concise definition of management. Management is working with and through individuals and groups to accomplish organizational goals. To be successful, organizations must require their management to have interpersonal skills. The achievement of organizational objectives through leadership is management.

While management and leadership are often considered the same thing, there is an important distinction. Leadership is a broader concept than management. Management is a special kind of leadership in which the achievement of the organization goals is paramount. The key difference is in the word *organization*. Leadership occurs any time one attempts to *influence the behavior* of an individual or group regardless of the reason. It may be for one's own goals or those of others, and they may or may not be congruent with organizational goals.

It is generally agreed that there are at least three areas of skill necessary for carrying out the process of management: technical, human, and conceptual. To be effective, less technical skill tends to be needed as one advances from lower to higher levels in an organization, but more and more conceptual skill is required. While the amount of technical and conceptual skill varies at different management levels, the common denominator that appears to be crucial at all levels is human skill.

The successful organization has one major attribute that sets itself apart from unsuccessful organizations: dynamic and effective leadership. Management texts by Peter F. Drucker (1964, 1967, 1973, 1980) are renowned for their insights and contributions to management and leadership behavior. But there are no unique characteristics or qualities that can be used to ascertain the effective leaders from the ineffective. What the literature shows is that leadership is a dynamic process, varying from situation to situation with changes in leaders, followers, and situations. Leadership behavior becomes the most significant element in ascertaining leadership capability.

There is a body of knowledge about human organizations that undergirds the practice of management. Sophisticated managers utilize the general theory to deal with the individual institution. It is a theory that informs a manager of diagnostic issues and action approaches. It is, at the same time, the uniqueness of each organization that informs a manager of specific problems in that organization and what actions can make a difference in its performance.

Managers have choices, a much greater range of choices than is generally recognized. In part, managers do not recognize the range of choices available because their knowledge and skills are limited. In part, some managers have trouble sorting out their individual desires from organizational potential and desire. Every organization has constraints, and every manager is accordingly constrained; but within these constraints, more options exist for improving organizational performance than are usually recognized. Managers can develop different strategies for dealing with the external environment and for managing each of the organization's subsystems and sets of interdependencies.

Management work is decision-making, in its broadest sense, addressed to the achievement of organizational performance. The scope of this work includes acquiring and deploying resources, and facilitating performance of work. Much of this work is addressed to identifying and solving organizational problems.

ISSUES AND DILEMMAS

It should be fairly clear that I have almost come full circle to the social work systems model approach I detailed earlier. Based on the frame of reference I came from, the role of manager and administrator came easier to me. However as a social work manager coming from a strong clinical experience with significant rewards through my interventions, the low yield of reward as a manager was a bit disconcerting. My successful role as a social work advocate within my hospital often became a handicap. In budget sessions, fighting for rational deployment of limited resources and trying to deal with a "bottom line" mentality, I was accused of being too emotional, a typical social worker, not having become a "true" administrator. More often than not, it was the nursing service administrator and I arguing with others regarding patient care.

The roughest transition was learning to postpone rewards and to look for long range goals and successes. The ambivalence was always present to return to clinical practice yet ultimately the challenge of trying to change my colleagues or affect change in the organization was the major reason I remained in management.

Regularly my administrative colleagues took shots at my participative style of problem solving, my knowledge and involvement in patient care issues. My assignment of course provided me with that access and gave me some sense of strength and power. However in budget interactions, the proof of my administrative skills was in the way I portrayed myself. It was a game of playing "hard nose," appearing callous, in order to gain acceptance. It was a real trap for me to avoid, yet often seductive in its quick access to acceptance. Becoming a manager within a setting where you were once a clinician may or may not be a blessing. Performance expectations are obviously different where they previously know you as opposed to not knowing you at all. Leadership style change may need to be more abrupt in the former case and not allow you to adapt to a style through a growth process. There's no real time for experimentation.

Within our organization, there was a significant status to having an MHA degree and preferably from one specific school. I periodically explored this avenue and sought out other opportunities as well. However, it was clear that the MHA was a stepping stone to further advancement. I chose an alternative route, however, gaining an advanced certificate in hospital administration which placated my more vocal critics. While only one quarter semester from an MHA, I have no real desire to complete it as my new position draws strongly from my social work community organization skills and my human behavior skills. My desire for further education or knowledge now is focused on learning about public policy, strategic planning, and strategic management.

Looking more closely at my past manager role has also caused me to look at leadership issues. The old self-determination plaudit becomes an impediment where certain management decisions have to be made. The ideal of involving your employees or staffs in the decision-making process is not often a reality, yet hopefully you know enough of where your staff is at that the decision, particularly if it affects them more distinctly, is more acceptable. We know decisions can't be made in a vacuum but you will regularly see it happen from a manager who lacks good human skills. I found it valuable to do some reading on leadership and leadership styles to get to know myself better, to learn to adjust my style to situations, and remain sensitive to the issues. That sensitivity can be drawn upon at later times when the issue of a decision is less emotionally laden.

Similarly, gaining greater insight into the various kinds of power one can have, how to use them or not use them, and to recognize a specific power type where used on you, added immeasurably to my working within the organization. Power does not necessarily beget success—it may only provide temporary compliance—until the "next time." Then, watch out!

Within management as well, is the whole concept of effectiveness and efficiency. I discussed some of this earlier but suffice it to say that there is a major difference between "getting things done right" and "getting the right things done." Too often we get trapped into the former approach as managers. Managers have lots of choices and our social work skills of diagnosis, plan, and treatment, should assist us to accomplish the right things.

As the whole health care scene changes, it is important that we broaden our understanding of financial management, strategic planning, and marketing. These additional skills are our survival paths (Peters and Waterman, 1982). Social work is a soft service, yet the good manager can put hard value to its services from a financial perspective. The literature is already filled with examples. Strategic planning skills are equally significant not only in positioning your social work program effectively within your organization but also placing its expertise and contribution at the disposal of the organization as part of its (the organization's) positioning process. That takes knowledge and skill, an awareness of the total goals of the institution, and where you can be most effective and useful.

In my new position, I draw regularly from my experiences and my educational resources. I've experienced both positive and negative management situations, have even contributed to their success and failure. However, the experiences have been good learning situations and have provided me with a measure of strength and self confidence which has enabled me to make some critical professional personal decisions regarding my future. It goes without saying that these experiences have enabled me to also be an effective corporate director, an efficient manager, and a creative leader—and that's what makes my job *fun!*

IMPLICATIONS

What does all this mean for social work practice, education, and research and study? In my mind, it is critical that social work needs to provide a strong generic base of practice so that as each practitioner explores various career challenges. Basic skills must be entrenched and one can draw from that depth of knowledge as you move in your career and feel confident in that knowledge as decisions are made. That a social worker builds upon that generic base to become a clinical specialist is not a critical issue. To build upon that base to become a manager or an executive is significantly more important.

Remembering some of my social work administration courses, I recall that they were setting specific, i.e., public welfare, health setting, private/public social agency. I feel that a broader perspective needs to be taught to provide more basic skills and knowledge about management as a profession and a means to effective leadership. Organizational behavior and management of organizations are important knowledge elements to have a mastery of before embarking naively into the foray. Clinicians do not always make good managers but one must know what makes a good manager. Assessment of what your strengths and weaknesses are in light of management requirements or skills is important. It is easy to move up without thinking about what changes may be necessary. It's a great ego booster to be chosen by your leaders for an elevated position. The money might be a significant incentive as well. Both are superficial sirens.

As social workers are afforded more opportunities to assume non-social work administrative positions, research would seem indicated to focus on why the organization leadership chose that person. What assets, behaviors, skills were significant and over time, were those judgements validated through employee performance. What factors were weakest, what skills were less important later than earlier might be areas to assess. Comparative studies with social work administrators would lend additional insight and knowledge to the whole management field. Evaluating the forces of economic pressures, leaner times, and the impact of less altruistic approaches to decision making on the social worker turned non-social work administrator as against "better times" would make interesting information. This could be expanded to looking at the frequency of social worker elevation to administration in hard times versus good times and why it occurs or doesn't.

Regardless of what social work practice eventually comes to, what education finally develops for students of management, what research and study extracts from its information, management and administration are extreme challenges. Yet I feel social workers have the best background and talent from which to build solid management and leadership skills. Regardless of the setting, you have to get the right things done to be an effective and efficient manager. What a terrific challenge—and it's fun!

REFERENCES

Charns, Martin P. and Schaefer, Margarite J. *Health Care Organization: A Model for Management.* Prentice-Hall, Inc., Englewood Cliffs, N.J., 1983.
Drucker, Peter F. *The Practice of Management,* Harper and Row: New York, 1973.
———, *The Effective Executive.* Harper and Row: New York, 1967.

_____, *Managing for Results*, Pan Publishing Co.: London, 1964.

_____, *Managing in Turbulent Times*, Harper and Row: New York, 1980.

Hersey, Paul and Blanchard, Ken. *Management of Organizational Behavior: Utilizing Human Resources*, Fourth Edition., Prentice-Hall, Inc.: Englewood Cliffs, N.J., 1982.

Peters, Thomas J. and Waterman, Robert H. *In Search of Excellence*. Harper and Row Publishers: New York, 1982.

Pincus, Allen and Minahan, Anne. *Social Work Practice: Model and Method*. F. D. Peacock Publishers, Inc., Itasca, Illinois, 1973.

CHAPTER VIII

The Social Worker as Manager in Health Care Settings: An Experiential View

Gary Rosenberg, PhD

As I examine my experiences as a social worker and as a hospital manager, I shall try to be as objective as possible, given that these are subjective experiences. My concern is for accuracy in describing issues, dilemmas and conflicts as they occurred at the time, as they seemed to me in retrospect and how I now look at these events with a perspective influenced by time.

CURRENT POSITION AND RESPONSIBILITIES

My current position at this large, urban medical center with a 1100 bed hospital and a medical school covers three areas of responsibility. I am a corporate Vice President; the Director of The Department of Social Work Services; and Professor of Community Medicine (Social Work).

Vice President for Human Resources

In this capacity I am responsible for (1) the development of health policy for the medical center's multiple programs of patient care services and (2) for the management of the "human resource" function, the new concept used for describing activities clustered around the employees of an organization.

The health policy function covers the medical center's relationship with the local community as well as with those with municipal, state and federal agencies in relation to health affairs. In the first, the goal is to

71

understand and better meet the health care needs of the residents of our local community of East Harlem. In the second, the goal is to understand and influence the impact of legislation on the center's ability to serve patients and preserve economic viability.

The term "human resource" is one which tries to replace the bureaucratic processing connotation of "personnel departments" with the concept that an organization's most valuable assets are the individuals who work for it. In the human resource function, I am responsible for the major personnel functions of most organizations, with the exception of labor relations: for recruitment and employment for the hospital and the medical school; systems of compensation and benefits; programs of orientation, affirmative action and training of management/supervisory personnel; design and maintenance of personnel records; recreation for staff and medical students; and organizational development.

In addition to the Department of Human Resources itself many other "human" resource departments are responsible and report directly to me:

Social Work
Government Relations
Community Relations
Patient Advocacy (Patient Representative Department)
Volunteer Department
Applied Social Research (marketing studies)

With the exception of Social Work, where I retain the position of Director, each of these departments has its own director.

In addition to these line management responsibilities, I carry staff responsibility for several Board of Trustee Committees including the Auxiliary Board, The Community and Government Affairs Committee, the Public Affairs Committee and the Compensation Committee. I also assist, along with the Director of the Hospital, in staffing its Patient Care Committee whose function is to monitor quality of patient care, particularly staff behaviors and attitudes, and consumer satisfaction.

My direct reporting responsibility is to the President of the Medical Center. I also work closely with the Dean of the Medical School and the Director of the Hospital, with a direct reporting relationship to the last for Social Work.

Director, Department of Social Work Services

Here I carry the classical responsibilities for the management of the social work department and its 100 plus staff in our service, education and research functions.

Professor of Community Medicine (Social Work)

Here I perform educational and research activities in the Medical School for medical students and students of allied health professions including social work on masters and doctoral levels.

This is an exciting combination of responsibilities connected with multiple systems within and outside the institution: external systems of national and state health policy and those in the local community; in house systems of patient care, human resource management, organizational development, medical center education and research. Managing and influencing these systems tap a spectrum of interpersonal and organizational skills, and multilevelled layers of specialized knowledge.

THE TRANSITION TO CURRENT RESPONSIBILITIES

My career at the Medical Center began 9 years ago as Associate Director of the hospital's social work department. From the beginning, the responsibilities fanned out beyond the department to include kindred functions. I had the concurrent appointment to the medical school and its concomitant education and research responsibilities; I was responsible for the management of the patient advocacy (Patient Representative) department, a service which the previous social work leader helped develop and implement; of the Department of Volunteers; and for the role of consultant to the Auxiliary Board which carries significant educational and service functions in the center.

Thus, from the onset, my work here straddled the systems of service delivery, management, education and research, spanning both the hospital and medical school organizations. Soon after I arrived, the director of the hospital asked me to take on a number of hospital wide projects. For example, I was asked to chair a committee of neonatologists in Pediatrics and Obstetrics whose purpose was to achieve a rational and helpful organization of care for neonates and to better coordinate the education of residents in prenatal and neonatal care. This involved working to resolve proprietary vested interests of each of these departments: of keeping a balanced focus on the needs of the medical center, of the needs of patients and of the teaching and service needs, in a background of competition with other medical centers who had a similar goal to develop feeder hospitals in order to become a regional neonatal center. This work required interpersonal skills, the ability to relate to all sides of an issue and with all the people who took these sides. In other words, it needed a capacity to deal with constructive conflict. Conflict did not scare me as it was part of my training and experience as a clinician and therapist. I also understood that problem resolution comes about through process and although we are not always clear about outcome, social workers know a lot about process.

The successful completion of such difficult management tasks brought recognition of my administrative capability by hospital management, and a reputation for being able to resolve difficult interdepartmental and human relations issues which in turn led to my appointment to the Senior Management Team of the hospital.

As I reflect on these events, I see these dynamics operating. The department's long tradition of innovation and excellence in the delivery of social work service, research and education, and its strong leadership over a period of 35 years contributed consistently and incrementally to the positive view of social work held by important constituencies in the medical center. Over these years, the department developed strong allies and supporters including chairman of medical departments, some managers, the Auxiliary Board (the department's original sponsor), members of the Board of Trustees, members of the medical school faculty who thought it important enough to extablish a Division of Social Work, and donors who established a professional chair for social work in the medical school, the first and perhaps the only such in the country.

The department's history and its visibility in both the hospital and the medical school are significant factors in the emergence of opportunities which broadened the sphere of my responsibilities. I think these opportunities arose as much because of that history as because of my particular talents. Where social work departments have established positive visibility and influence in an institution there is a likelihood that such opportunities will develop.

But it is also true that my abilities were known to the Director of the hospital as we had worked together previously at another hospital. Also, the institution was looking for individuals with a systems approach who at the same time could care for individuals *and* manage resources. These projects were a way of testing my aptitudes.

I was motivated to take on new responsibilities. I was "ambitious," if you like. I always expanded my responsibilities into areas new to me and moved into roles of clinician, educator, student, manager, etc., simultaneously. I enjoyed the excitement of new challenges. But most important, I felt there was an opportunity to demonstrate the profession's usefulness in health care management in a broadened and expanded way (Rosenberg and Weissman, 1981). And the additional compensation was certainly important to a (gourmet) father of four.

As noted, my work on these projects helped make my system skills and commitment to people visible to other members of the hospital senior management team. My ability to straddle and operate with comfort in the three systems of clinical social work delivery in the hospital, hospital management and the academic medical school added to my credibility with these colleagues as I joined them as a member.

The Senior Management Team, which directs the operation of the hospital, is a matrix organization.

On its horizontal axis are those managers, most of whom are vice presidents (I was not one) who control the institution's resources—its personnel, materials, spaces, and finances. These managers include the directors of nursing, support services, personnel, and finance. On the vertical axis are the physician-managers who control the institution's programs—typically separated into Medicine, Surgery, Psychiatry, etc. The importance of the program dimension in management is particularly relevant in teaching institutions, where the actions of full-time medical staff directly influence the use of the hospital's resources.

At this hospital we have implemented the program-resource concept, a form of matrix organization. Under this system of management, almost every hospital employee serves two designated "masters," one for program function and one for resource function. This allows the hospital employee to have dual identification (Davis and Carswell, 1977). For example, through the program resource concept, social work is able to identify not only as a member of the program department, (i.e., renal dialysis) but simultaneously as a member of the social work profession (i.e., the social work department). Similarly, other health resource personnel are able to identify both with their professions and with their treatment teams.

The basic functions of a resource-department head are to recruit and hire personnel, train them in the discipline of the department, assign them to program responsibilities, supervise their work within the discipline, evaluate and promote them within the discipline, and dismiss those whose performance is unsatisfactory. The resource-department head also serves as a consultant in his/her discipline to the other program directors.

While resource-department heads have responsibility for setting objectives that relate to their own disciplines and for the resources for which they are responsible, program directors also are able to function effectively under a system of management by objectives. Each program director must develop a general statement of objectives for their program. The measure of their performance is how well they achieve stated objectives. If resources are committed to the program consistent with those objectives, they are obliged to carry out the objectives. If resources cannot be committed, they may reduce the scope and content of program objectives. Thus, the program-resource concept establishes a clear basis for organizational accountability and the development of measures of performance (Rosenberg, 1980).

Basically, the program resource concept requires the ability not to be cornered by either of the two masters, to be comfortable in arguing principle and in excluding it, to be at the same time client centered and institution centered.

Since the basic task of the medical center in 1978 was to move to a break even financial position in order to submit a certificate of need to rebuild the hospital and to enter the debt market with a break-even performance, the majority of senior management meetings focused on financial management in relation to programs and priorities. I needed to learn a great deal more about financial management in order to effectively participate as a member of the Senior Management Team. To become better prepared in financial management skills, I took advanced coursework at a graduate school of business.

By the end of 1980, we had achieved a break-even position without the use of depreciation funds. At that time, the President of the hospital began a major organizational development effort to enhance behaviors and attitudes of personnel, to rearrange the organization of the institution so it could deliver compassionate care to match the high technical level of its quality medical care. After an intensive search for someone to manage and lead this organizational development effort, I was asked if I would consider a position which separated labor relations (as an advisory function) from the human resource concern for the employee, the work environment, the organization and its missions. Given my performance as a senior manager, my previous background working in organizational development including a doctorate in the sociology of complex organizations and the sociology of health care, and the credibility I developed with physicians in the clinical and academic departments, I was offered the position of Vice President for Human Resources with the primary task of working on organizational development issues (Beckhard and Harris, 1977; Margulies and Adams, 1982). Specifically, we set as our goal to revitalize the spirit and substance of the service ethic throughout the Medical Center and to create an organizational climate in which:

— Patients would perceive the hospital as a warm, caring, friendly and efficient institution where personnel at all levels are courteous, competent and compassionate.

— Physicians, nurses and other professionals would perceive the services of the hospital as supportive of their therapeutic management of their patients.

— All personnel would identify with the purposes of the Medical Center; show concern and compassion for patients and cooperation with fellow workers; develop the skills necessary to meet high standards of performance; and display initiative and creativity in carrying out day-to-day activities.

— The institution would provide for its employees: (a) incentives which encourage solid performance and increase opportunities for self-worth, growth and satisfaction in the workplace; (b) a total compensation approach with a systematic approach to job classification and career-pathing; and (c) responsive, effective recruitment and selection processes (Speedling and Rosenberg, 1986).

I list these goals in some detail in order to highlight how neatly they fit into the concept of social work functions in regard to an organization's systems. In the ecological view, we see social work function as broader than direct services to the patient and family, and extending to include intervention and influence on the institution's ambience as it affects patient recovery. Because of their knowledge and skill in the processes of social change, social workers have much to offer to organizational development efforts. This was an opportunity to use these skills in a larger arena affecting the entire institution, both its employees and patients (Beckhard, 1969). The job needs matched my skill and training with people and systems. I believe it is not accidental that so many organizational efforts use social work input.

This initial offer included the request that I give up the directorship of the Social Work Department. This caused conflict within me which put me in touch with the deep, serious and abiding commitment to my chosen profession. I did not want to give that up. I doubt if I would have taken on the managerial work and liked it enough without the social work piece. Also, I had seen many excellent social workers move into management positions and give up the social work operation and I wanted to see if there was another way. It was an intellectual experiment as well as a personal one: can a social worker remain in social work and still exert influence as a manager? Too, I think retaining my social work position provided both a psychological as well as a realistic safety valve—in case it didn't work out, I'd still have my home base.

Management's concern about my retaining the social work department directorship was whether I could give enough time to both components. And this certainly was a valid concern in view of my already heavy schedule as a manager, therapist and teacher, with the multiple allied activities they entailed.

There was considerable negotiation back and forth. I was willing to think about giving up the leadership of the social work department but only if I was first permitted to try it with the package I wanted. Also, I kept making the case that in fact the two components were related, both in substance and in skill. Knowledge of patient needs is directly usable in any health care management job and particularly in organizational development efforts as well as in the management of human resources. And I think the hospital director finally considered it more responsible to leave me with a fall back position.

Thus, after much negotiation back and forth, it was agreed that I would remain Director of Social Work for a trial period of two years during which I also assumed the Vice Presidency of Human Resources and responsibility for the organizational development effort. Once that agreement was reached, two issues confronted me in this new position: (1) what would be the reaction of the department of social work, and the other departments accountable to me, and (2) how would the human resources personnel react to a change in leadership and the change in focus of their work.

The staff of the Department of Social Work Services reacted cautiously to my new responsibilities. They were concerned about whether I was committed to remain active as their director and if so would I have the time to devote to leadership in the department and to their needs. They were also, however, pleased that one of their number was selected to assume additional responsibilities in the medical center.

The reality was that I had to manage this enormous increase in responsibilities within the same extended work day without giving short shrift to any one component. I did this by paring, not eliminating activities. I gave up some of teaching responsibilities in schools of social work, and some of my outside speaking engagements. I reduced my committee work outside the hospital with the Society for Hospital Social Work Directors and other organizations. I cut my patient load to 10 hours per week. And I did give less time to the direct management of the social work department. This was possible because of the high caliber deputy director who took over the day to day operation of the department and manages it capably.

As far as the social workers' concern about my ability to stay related to their needs, I acknowledged that some of this was real and some might not be. I enunciated that I would always be there for issues of policy and program but openly admitted I had less time to spend directly with staff. I created a new organizational structure in the department so that programs are managed by top quality social work managers (assistant directors), to whom staff would relate. In essence, my operating responsibilities were pushed down one level. With the reorganization of the department and the structure weekly management meetings I chaired, I could still direct the overall operation and stay involved in policy and programs.

Members of the Department of Human Resources also had mixed feelings about their new vice-president. They were reassured by the fact that they would be represented with significant influence at the higher levels of medical center policy and decision making. They were concerned, however, about my lack of experience in human resource matters and about how quickly I would come to learn their needs and become an effective advocate for them.

Here I openly acknowledged what I did and did not know. I attended many conferences to learn more. I used staff input extensively and respectfully. It helped that I did not manage the department operations directly but that an efficient director did. And I did obtain additional resources for them which they had needed for some time. This clinched their view of me as effective.

While I had had experience in organizational change in smaller institutions, the magnitude of the task at this 1100 bed academic teaching hospital with an on site medical school, required, in my opinion as well as that of the Senior Management Team, help from a set of consultants which would allow me to carefully plan and implement the organizational development efforts. Two consultants were hired, one to deal with the general strategy of approaching the organizational issues and a second whose task was to implement the first part of our strategy which was built on an organizational diagnoses. Both these consultant relationships provided additional continuing education for me by updating me on the most recent theories and practice of organizational development and affording the opportunity to review those theories in a tutorial relationship (Beckhard, 1969).

There were other aspects of human resources with which I was far less familiar, such as affirmative action, benefits management, job classification systems, equitable and competitive cash compensation and the particular laws that govern a personnel department. In order to learn these I used the familiar strategy of reading, attending conferences, and taking courses. In a short period of time I was able to increase my knowledge in these areas. In pursuing these various avenues for increasing my knowledge, I felt comfortable in acknowledging where I lacked expertise and embarked on these programs without feelings of inadequacy.

During the two year trial period I was able to demonstrate successful leadership with the dual focus and the arrangement has continued to date.

In 1985, a new president of the medical center added Government and Community Relations to my responsibilities. I was more adequately prepared for both of these two additional functions, given my background in sociology and social work.

SOCIAL WORK MANAGEMENT EXPERIENCE

The history of social work is replete with references to the need for greater specialization in management skills. One author, summarizing the emergence of administrative and management skills in social work, suggested that "by the 1950s it was apparent that administration was becoming an inherent part of the whole social work process rather than merely a tool, adjunct or facilitating device" (Patti, 1983). Between the 50s and 70s not enough was done to promote social work management skills. In the early 70s, Rosemary Saari (1973) warned social work educators that:

> Unless the profession demonstrates that it can meet critical social needs . . . and provide leadership in the design and delivery of social services, it will be relegated to roles as private practitioners and handmaidens to other professions. . . . Schools must prepare individuals to be able to enter the socio/political arena at all levels of government to succeed in the planning, design, implementation and evaluation of effective services.

In order to describe my experiences in social work management and how they influenced my current roles and responsibilities it is important to place them in the context of social work management in the profession over the years of my development. The experience in the 70s and 80s and even in the late 60s demonstrated that Saari was correct in her predictions. More social programs were placed under the influence of attorneys and business managers, particularly high level policy positions. In the 80s, joint programs developed between schools of social work and schools of business and post graduate programs in social work administration were available to the interested practitioner or manager.

The special nature of social work management has been described by many scholars (Patti, 1983; Saari and Hasenfeld, 1978). Among the most relevant to my experiences is *societal ambivalence to the need for administrative advocacy* (Patti, 1983). Social work administrators cannot always assume a stable, continuing base of socio/political support and one must ordinarily devote considerable effort to winning support for department and goals for patient care. This is particularly true in the health care setting where support for social work services, which are so often viewed as a "guest" service, must be weighed against the financial contingencies of the hospital's income, assets and expenses. Gaining this support has become a critical skill. The successful social work departments have been those which have understood how to mesh the goals of department advocacy and the goals of the medical center. This includes the ability to delay advocacy or attempt to frame advocacy for patients and for the social work department in terms congruent with the organization, wherever possible. Too many social work directors believe that doing what is "right" is the only way of thinking about things; and doing what is "right" is perceived only in light of how the social work director perceives it and not others in the organization. This leads to a negative reaction to what social work has to say and contribute. It is important to avoid this perception by others. One can identify oneself with the point of view of the department, and with the point of view of the patients it serves, particularly the disadvantaged or those in need of care, but always within a framework of understanding the conflicting needs of the organization as well as the organization's priorities and value system.

In order to create receptivity to program expansion and refinement, social work managers must also work to modify attitudes regarding the client groups they serve and alter the stereotypes about how to deal with such clients. The client groups which social work serves in health care settings vary. The definitions of risk and needs frequently apply to the wealthy as well as to the poor, and thus social work can advocate not only for the disadvantaged but for those in need, regardless of economic circumstance. Social work advocacy must be framed within the values and ethics of the profession, but with an understanding that frequently what we advocate for, particularly with regard to the disadvantaged, is not always in the perceived interest of the medical center and those who manage it. Respect for that perception is the best way to change it. Broad based advocacy is important in that it helps administrators who would otherwise conveniently pigeon-hole us into advocating only for the disadvantaged and downtrodden, to perceive our advocacy as more broadly-based and, as frequently as possible, linked with missions and goals of the organization.

Social work administrators need to contribute to the overall understanding of the organization's efforts and goals so that these do not violate or threaten widely held community values and norms (Patti, 1983). A major dimension of social work management skills is the ability to support and cooperate in an environment of diverse expectations. Social work managers work in a complex environment and need to maintain contact with diverse constituencies; when they keep abreast of changing needs and circumstances they can translate these to the organization in an effective way. In working with different constituencies we provide a common base of understanding for psychosocial services in a framework of mutual respect and understanding. The clinical application of collaboration skills are transferable to the management of health care social work services. These same clinical collaborative skills must be translated into systems collaboration, that is, collaboration with key constituencies in and outside of the medical center. While social work's power base is frequently collaborative it is also formed on service strategies which also require extensive collaborative skills. Attempts at broad-based collaboration on the management level are frequently met with distrust, particularly if the management style is that of everyone fighting for what they need and want, and of protecting their departments rather than dealing with the greater good of the organization. When the management style is one that puts organizational goals before departmental ones which only affect some departments rather than the institution as a whole, then collaboration can be viewed as an asset. Collaboration does not necessarily minimize conflict but puts conflict in a framework which allows for resolution in the interest of the organization.

These dimensions are the ones that I found particularly germane and useful in the responsibilities that I now carry. In addition, there were certain management skills and tasks which are part of every good social work director's armamentarium of skills, including program planning, the creation of new programs, financial management and the demonstration of social work's efficiency and effectiveness to the organization (Rosenberg, 1980). Social work brings a systems focus for problem-solving, a focus on the individual patient (the client system) and on the system of care (policy and programs). This focus is useful, applicable and transferable to management functions and tasks; and it enhances primary management skills.

The last skill which I will discuss is leadership. Leadership qualities are crucial in the transition from clinician to social work manager and also in the transition from social work manager to hospital manager. American organizations have been over-managed and under-led (Peters and Waterman, 1982). Leadership in social work in health care requires a capacity to be fair, participate equitably with workers and other management staff in decision making; to collaborate with respect for and understanding of human behavior and systems; to encourage creativity, reward program innovation, believe in personal excellence and be able to communicate a sense of belief in people's capacities, values and entitlements.

I believe there were certain personal characteristics which helped me be a good social work manager and also in the transition to hospital management. These characteristics include a love for adventure. Being a manager is not just a job, it is a personal commitment. It takes tenacious preparation and requires a great deal of self-respect and courage. One must have a passion for excellence and one must be optimistic and communicate that optimism even during difficult times (Peters and Austin, 1985).

One must work hard and be ambitious, ambitious for one's personal ends but also for the social values that one believes in. Working hard includes reading about what you do not know, keeping up with the literature; if you have multiple tasks and multiple responsibilities, it means keeping up with more literature, attending more conferences, learning by teaching and learning by doing. Another important talent is creativity, the ability not to be constrained by usual ways of thinking, but to look for new and innovative ways of doing things.

CONCLUSION

Social work training and experience are not in and of themselves a prerequisite for hospital management. There are, however, certain aspects of social work which are useful in hospital management. They include direct contact with patients, an appreciation of client systems, appreciation of the perspective of the consumer in looking at services, commitment to and skill in collaborative practice, knowledge and skill in group dynamics; values which include and appreciate all levels of personnel and their contributions; understanding the social effects of interventions on individuals, groups, communities and management; comfort in dealing with conflict.

Planning, managing and controlling functions are not ones which are taught in schools of social work. Financial management, personnel management skills, being responsible for the bottom line, and organizational change and development are all aspects of management which are not inherently part of social work nor do I think they should be a major part of social work curriculum. Any social worker wishing to move into hospital management will need additional education and perhaps additional degrees to be successful.

Another requirement includes personal capabilities. Here social workers are not unlike others in that some are demonstrably more capable of moving ahead than others. Some wish to move ahead and others do not. Then there are the set of personal characteristics which are useful in the transition from social work manager to hospital manager. The need of the organization, how the organization and its leadership perceive social work and the particular social worker in quest of larger responsibilities, and the timeliness of what that social worker has to offer are important factors in moving into management. From my own experience I think that all of these are necessary ingredients. For myself I would not give up the social work function. I suppose one does not realize the importance of one's commitment until the commitment itself is tested. Social workers who are now part of the management of health care can offer much to others in social work settings, to non-social work managers and members of management teams. The process of health care delivery requires as much empathy for the patient and understanding of the patient system as it does the understanding of financial planning, organizational development and care of the physical environment.

Managers in health care can assist in creating a therapeutic health care environment by helping staff and patients to predict and control what will happen to them, help preserve privacy, decrease social isolation, buffer patients and families from the threatening elements of the environment and encourage the comforting of patients and families.

Because patient/family needs are not confined within the boundaries of any single discipline or department, patients are served best when care is delivered with an interdisciplinary design. Health care cannot be delivered piecemeal, as if patients' needs were discrete and separate. Managers can take the lead in fostering a team approach to hospital care by affirming their *own* role in helping patients reach their potential for wellness; and by opening dialogues with clinical colleagues on the paramount subject of their *mutual* interest and responsibility: patient wellbeing.

REFERENCES

Beckhard, Richard. *Organizational Development, Strategies and Models,* Addison-Wesley: Massachusetts, 1969.

Beckhard, Richard and Harris, Ruben T. *Organizational Transitions: Managing Complex Change,* Addison-Wesley: Massachusetts, 1977.

Davis, Samuel and Carswell, W. "The Program Resource Concept: A Management Approach for an Academic Medical Center," *The Mount Sinai Journal of Medicine,* Vol. 4(5), September-October 1977, pp. 624–632.

Margulies, Newton and Adams, John B. *Organizational Development in Health Care Organizations,* Addison-Wesley: Massachusetts, 1982.

Patti, Rino J. *Social Welfare Administration,* Prentice Hall: N.J., 1983.

Peters, Tom and Austin, Nancy. *A Passion for Excellence: The Leadership Difference,* Random House, Inc.: N.Y., 1985.

Peters, Thomas J. and Waterman, Robert H. *In Search of Excellence,* Harper and Row: New York, 1982.

Rosenberg, Gary. "Concepts in Financial Management of Hospital Social Work Departments," *Social Work in Health Care,* Vol. 3, Spring 1980, pp. 287–297.

Rosenberg, Gary and Weissman, Andrew. "Marketing Social Services in Health Care Facilities," *Health and Social Work,* Vol. 6, August 1981, pp. 13–20.

Saari, Rosemary, "Effective Social Work Intervention in Administration and Planning Roles: Implications for Education, Facing the Challenge," New York Council on Education, 1973, p. 37.

Saari, Rosemary and Hasenfeld, Yeheskel. *The Management of Human Services,* Columbia University Press, New York, 1978.

Speedling, Edward J. and Rosenberg, Gary. "Patient Well-Being: A Responsibility for Hospital Managers," *Health Care Management Review,* Volume 11, No. 3, Summer, 1986, pp. 9–20.

CHAPTER IX

Philosophical Perspective on Social Work Administration

W. June Simmons, LCSW

INTRODUCTION

This chapter explores key issues in social work administration in a hospital setting. It is predicated on the assumption that an important social work responsibility in hospitals is to work to influence and infuse the hospital system with social work values and perspectives, a concept especially crucial in the current context of rapid redesign of the health care system. One method for achieving this objective is through the promotion of the social work director to a hospital administrative position. This represents a form of assimilation of social work into the hospital power structure and planning system.

In order to reach the stage of assimilation, I have found it is essential for the social work administrator to demonstrate a strong capacity for department leadership. I believe it important to select a theoretical practice perspective to serve as a focus and guide for the leadership of the social work department. The ecological systems perspective has guided my practice at Huntington Memorial Hospital. In implementing that theory, I gave particular attention to the development of consensus concerning the mission of social work as it interfaces with the hospital's changing mission. I worked collaboratively within the department, the hospital, and the community to achieve that mission.

Inherent in the Director's leadership role is bringing a clear philosophical base and a vision of a positive future for social work which can be achieved through setting standards of excellence, and by building a work

The author thanks Dr. Helen Northen for editing this chapter.

85

environment characterized by hope, persistence, and fairness. I found that with accurate assessment of the hospital's evolving readiness for the contributions that social work can make, and with interventions directed to demonstrating the social work contribution, a department may indeed gradually gain status and ultimately become assimilated into the upper power structure of the hospital.

CURRENT POSITION AND RESPONSIBILITIES

My current position is as Director of the Senior Care Network and the Patient Services Department (Clinical Social Work). Twenty-five percent of my time is spent in planning, financial management and program consultation with the social work department director and its management team. Seventy-five percent of my time is spent in directing the Senior Care Network. This position reports directly to the Vice President of Administration for the hospital and is connected to the Board of Directors through its Senior Care Council, a fund raising and advisory board which is chaired by the Vice Chairman of the Board.

This position is a hospital administrative post which requires the essential perspective of the social work administrator to assure that the redesign of the health system is clinically sound. Financial management, interpersonal skills entailed in planning, introducing major institutional change, and community networking are key capabilities.

While the new position represents a significant promotion and advancement into hospital administration, it is also designed to retain my direct involvement in the social work department. This is an intentional approach reflecting the philosophy that promotion of the social work director should result in elevation of the social work department itself. The social work patient care perspective is an important balance needed in health care planning today. I believe this contribution cannot be made if the social work director leaves the direct line to the profession and its understanding and knowledge of the patient's experience. I think this is an essential viewpoint for the design of today's newly emerging health care delivery system. This joint direction assures ongoing social work leadership in the new program directions and links discharge planning and community-based care for optimum continuity.

In following this model, I found the losses that accompany promotion are minimized. Given a strong internal social work management structure that can take on a stronger role, the transition entailed shifts in my key leadership functions and roles. The Associate Director assumed Department Head status in social work, assuming primary management of department operations. But my key relationships within the department itself and my direct involvement in major issues, direction-setting, and problem-solving are ongoing, although I am inevitably more involved in a wider range of activities outside social work.

THE TRANSITION

Career transitions occur in the context of the host organization and its historical roots. So too, my current position is best viewed in that context. Huntington Memorial Hospital is a 606 bed private non-profit acute hospital located in Pasadena, California. The medical center is well-managed, well-financed and has a long standing teaching program which was originally free-standing and is currently affiliated with the University of Southern California School of Medicine. The hospital was founded in 1892 and is surrounded by and serves a remarkably diverse set of neighborhoods with a rich array of socio-economic status and ethnic diversity among the residents.

Social Work Department Beginnings

The growth of this hospital is relatively recent. In the late 1960s it was a small community hospital with less high technology and a conservative and homogeneous medical staff. The institution shifted its mission to become a major regional medical center. It has since then tripled in size, acquired an array of medical technologies and many new specialists to direct focused specialty programs. After the initial spurt of growth, the hospital, alerted by the Joint Commission on Accreditation that it was required to have social work services, hired me as its first MSW Director. Thus, in 1972 I began as a brand new Social Work Director in a hospital brand new to social work which has subsequently developed a full-service Department of Clinical Social Work. Moving to a mid-size department with supervisors heading up specialty care-giving teams in particular hospital programs has been a major transition. That gradual growth was driven by my management philosophy that client needs and financial viability of the host setting are the two single most important creative tensions driving the design of the high quality clinical care system.

Beginning with a staff of only myself and a full time secretary, we began by building on the social work functions already in existence at the hospital. A Bachelor's-level Director had managed a two staff department responsible for the charitable assistance program and providing some limited information, referral and discharge planning services. This office worked closely with the hospital's teaching clinics and primarily served patients with limited financial means.

I was employed to develop a professional social work program for the hospital with the assumption that some limited additional staffing resources might be necessary. Initially, one additional FTE was planned, someone well acquainted with the community and able to assist us in outreach to middle and upper income segments of our patient population.

Hospital administration thought these new services could serve some of their immediate needs. The hospital had recently expanded in size from 220 to 565 beds. Its reputation in the community rested on its strong positive personalized care services as well as the excellence of its medical staff. It was hoped that the new social work department, by adding an extra dimension of services to private pay patient care, and by tracking changes in the hospital system, could assist the hospital in sustaining this positive and personalized approach to patient care.

Developing Social Work Services

No one at the hospital had strong ideas about what the social work department should be or could be. Moving from an evolutionary, gradual developmental perspective, we worked closely with administration, nursing, physicians and our patients to collaboratively identify the actual needs for social work services and to begin to develop these in areas that wanted them. Our involvement in the charitable funds rooted us in financial counseling services. This was fortuitous as it put us in the positive position of having a concrete and valuable product for the hospital. Our approval was required in order to pay for hospital-based services from the sizeable charitable funds.

In an effort to preserve these funds, we became experts in assisting patients in first pursuing other entitlements and eligibilities. Our close relationship with the Business Office was educational and helped us frame our understanding of the patient experience in financial as well as clinical terms. Close alliance with this section of the hospital helped tune us in to important issues such as impacting the number of days in accounts receivables and helping the hospital maintain its Medicare waiver of liability. These were the cornerstones of our learning to identify clearly the financial value to hospital operations that resulted from our clinical interventions.

Inheriting responsibility for discharge planning services for the patients cared for in the teaching program, we expanded these services to all patients. In-depth collaboration with nursing resulted in strong nursing support at all levels; and ultimately, nursing helped to integrate nursing discharge planners into the social work department staff. Most of these services were centered in general medical/surgical floors. Moving from this traditional base, and seeking to demonstrate our capabilities through actual provisions of services rather than general descriptions, we began to move into provision of assessment, mental health services, teaching, consultation and personal support to hospital employees.

In surveying the environment for areas that wanted expanded social work services, we found a warm welcome in the Emergency Room where the chief physician and head nurse had a special interest in patient advocacy and a more comprehensive view of patients, including their psychological and social needs. Following the pattern of working by referral, we developed a style of expanding where there was real interest in our services. As the hospital itself began to develop and specialize, we found it was easiest to have social work to grow slowly and gradually in more traditional areas, and to introduce social work in a more formal way in brand new programs where nothing had existed before. The Neonatal Intensive Care Unit and Pediatric Cardiology Programs were the first such specialty programs. Soon the hospital medical staff decided to develop a rehabilitation program and later a cardiac rehabilitation program. Obtaining a seat in the planning groups for these programs, which are natural users of social work services, allowed us to articulate appropriate social work roles and build on external hospital standards for practice and staffing.

Expanding in each of these areas as the host services grew, social work is now mandated for a complete complement of social work roles as described later, and supports a caseload standard of one worker for every twelve patients in these specialty areas. Emergency Room practice grew steadily, but incrementally, finally resulting in 7-day coverage on both the day and evening shifts, with night coverage as needed. As these services developed over time, we eventually evolved to a sufficiency of staff and program complexity to garner support for full time social work supervisors in the rehabilitation, maternal child health and ambulatory care areas. Medicine/surgery, critical care and oncology are grouped into a fourth team with their own supervisor, who later became the Department's Associate Director and is now its current Department Head.[*]

As we began, we agreed that each staff member and volunteer was a strong and essential player in the development of the service, helping shape its form and functions. Beginning with a clear philosophy of change, we fully expected that most people would not want social work services or have a good understanding of how to utilize them initially. And we were convinced that we were faced with a 5–10 year effort to develop an adequate understanding and utilization of social work services throughout the medical center. This has proved to be a correct projection.

Ultimately developing a high quality, broadly defined clinical social work program with multiple specialities and reasonably adequate staffing, we moved into the area of outpatient services as we saw the health care system begin to redesign itself. Early efforts included the development of a biofeedback program, followed by building a medically-related psychotherapy service and moving ultimately to obtaining small program

[*]Neena Bixby

development grants and contracts in home care social work and for consultation with other hospitals. These efforts led to our current experience of recent extremely rapid growth with the funding by a large bequest for a program proposal described below; which was then followed by a series of private grants and larger contracts as we became a national model planning team and program development center in hospital-initiated geriatric services. This new program and department is called the Senior Care Network. Strong community networking efforts in collaborative health planning were natural outgrowths of our client centered practice; these pushed us always towards new program development and innovations in a collaborative planning process with other hospital disciplines and key community agencies.

Planning for a Model Program

In 1983, the Robert Wood Johnson Foundation proposed to fund 10 hospital-initiated long-term care model programs. Our department had received a few small grants previously, but this was our first occasion to seek large, outside funding for major program dreams of long standing in our clinical services teams. Writing that proposal offered an excellent opportunity for the social work department to engage in a collaborative discourse with key hospital managers about the future directions of the hospital in care of the elderly. Although we had not written a major grant request before, for years staff had noted needed changes in the system and had addressed those programatically wherever possible.

Based on what we saw at the bedside, our clinical and management staff had profound concerns about the elderly. We had concerns about hospitalized patients whose deterioration in health could have been preventable. We had a long standing desire to assist patients and their families avoid placement in skilled nursing facilities; and we were eager to build a mechanism for comprehensive assessment, coordination of care in the community and a way to build in missing programs that would sustain independence and care in the home. The effort to write this major grant placed us in important planning conversations with the Vice President of Medical Affairs, key administrators, including an Associate Administrator with shared values and concerns, and the leaders of the financial system of the hospital. We also worked closely with Public Relations, Community Development, the Volunteer Office, Rehabilitation Services and other interested members of the hospital team. This planning process developed our thinking, helped us articulate patient needs and new program ideas clearly, and garnered enthusiasm and support from the medical staff, hospital administration and key management leaders. While writing this major proposal was a difficult task, the fact that it forced a planning process focused by the external criteria of the

Robert Wood Johnson Foundation RFP, and tempered by the requirement of meeting their deadlines, made it one of the most fruitful developmental processes we had ever engaged in. It helped to model social work as a leader helping the hospital to address important concerns.

Although we did not receive the Robert Wood Johnson funding, the planning process positioned us perfectly for future development. A major trust was formed by the estate of Margaret Bundy Scott; and Huntington was one of nine agencies named by this Trust to compete for 10 years for the proceeds of the Trust. The Trust required that the hospital propose innovative ideas true to the hospital's mission ideas that represented the kinds of ideal activities we would pursue if funding were available. Fortunately for the social work department, the process of planning for the Robert Wood Johnson grant had created a good deal of enthusiasm among key decision makers in the hospital for the development of coordinated care and health promotion programs. So when this new funding opportunity came along, high level advocacy was provided, especially by the Vice President of Medical Affairs[*] and the Associate Administrator responsible for the social work department. The Chief Executive Officer[**] and the Board of Directors as well as the Vice President of Finance all reached agreement that this was the ideal project to take forward. With assistance from the Director of the American Hospital Association's Office on Aging and Long Term Care,[***] we developed an expanded version of the Robert Wood Johnson proposal, developed in response to the question: How would we proceed if we could have optimum funding to develop the model national planning program for hospital initiated leadership to transform the way we deliver health services to the elderly?

The result was the creation in December, 1985 of the Senior Care Network of Huntington Memorial Hospital. This is a comprehensive geriatric services planning grant which has successfully obtained additional outside program development and implementation funding as well. A multi-disciplinary team of researchers and planners were brought together to transform the health delivery system for care of the elderly and chronically ill of all ages. The charge of the project is to produce a design which will provide improved health care at reduced costs through coordinated care (case management) and health promotion. The focus is on prevention through health education as well as intensive professional education to improve the practice of physicians, nurses and members of other key disciplines. The program works to maximize existing agency resources in the community through developing networks for coordinated health planning, with an improved data base. The availability of staff

[*] Dr. Gilbert Kipnis
[**] Mr. Kevin Hegarty
[***] Dr. William Read

education and technical assistance for hospital and community program development are vital. Gaps in the continuum of care locally are being identified and filled through coordinated community health planning. Access to needed resources, accompanied by appropriate assessment and follow-up, has been developed through building an ideal hospital-directed case management program, a life care planning program and a new health care delivery program. This comprehensive system, targeted at promoting health and reducing institutionally-based care through proper assessment and coordination, is intended to be financially self-sustaining at the end of the first three years. Development and expansion of this program grew from concepts and proposals organized by the social work department.

Growth of this magnitude occurred out of ability to allow and foster strength in staff. Reporting to an enabling administrative leader[*] for the last half of these years was critical to our success. Strong advocacy by the Vice President of Medical Affairs assisted us through many points where conflict could have emerged and damaged our growth process. Selection of a strong and talented staff and development of leaders in that group was key. Without the loyalty and close collaboration of the Associate Director and now Chief of Patient Services,[**] this process could not have unfolded in the same way. Development of loyal and talented supervisors was crucial. Success of this magnitude comes from supportive and fully trusted collaborators working at an evolutionary pace to make modest but cumulative changes over time; working toward a shared achievement with a positive vision of a hospital in which social work is an essential member with a strong and positive clinical team.

After 12 years of development, the social work department had 2 cost centers of its own and transferred costs to 4 other program centers, with a staff of 35 FTEs.

With the receipt of one bequest from the Margaret Bundy Scott Trust, and the addition of the new Senior Care Department in 1985–86, we essentially doubled in size.

The creation of the Senior Care Network resulted in my promotion to the direction of that program while I retained part-time administrative leadership within the social work department. The promotion of the Associate Director of the Social Work Department to Chief of the Department made it possible for us to retain our strength and quality within while accepting the vital opportunity for growth and expansion that social work direction of this model program would represent. At the end of the first year-and-a-half of successful operation, I was again promoted to the senior management team of the hospital.

---

[*] Gail Larsen
[**] Neena Bixby

SOCIAL WORK MANAGEMENT—A THEORETICAL FRAMEWORK

Professional practice is by definition directed by a theoretical frame-work. Social work practice in health care at Huntington Memorial Hospital takes direction from systems theory and the ecological perspective. This provides a client-centered focus, with multiple arenas of practice which build toward macro interventions. This guiding theoretical framework is best illustrated through the concentric circles illustrated in Figure 1.

The literature has only recently developed theoretical frameworks specific to social work practice in health care. Coulton (1979) outlines a useful perspective on the "fit" between person-environment as the focus in health care. She notes that substantial agreement seems to exist among social workers that the focus of social work is the person and environment in interaction; and that the profession's purpose is to promote or restore

Patient Care and Treating the Context of Patient Care

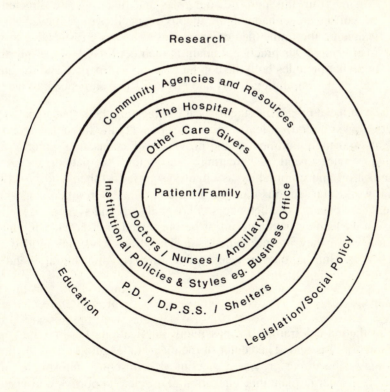

Figure 1

a mutually beneficial interaction between individuals and society. She further notes that "person-environment fit refers to the degree of congruence or correspondence between the individual's needs, capabilities, and aspirations, and the resources, demands and opportunities characteristic of the environment" (page 5). Her rationale is broader than that developed earlier by Pincus and Minahan (1973). Coulton points to a definition of social work practice that goes beyond direct counseling services for patients and families or providing direct resource-related services. Policy development is mandated. Systems interventions are requisite.

Coulton's view is compatible with the ecological perspective of Germain (1977) who notes that "The ecological perspective suggests that our social work purpose is to improve the quality of transactions between people and environments so there is a better match between people's adaptive potential and environmental qualities" (page 68). This mandate implies treating both the patient and organizational systems. As Germain states,

> Arising from this purpose, our roles and functions are directed to supporting and enhancing the adaptive capacities of people and to influencing the immediate environment to be more responsive to human needs. Our practice domain is then conceived as the interface area that includes both the coping behaviors of people and the qualities of the impinging social and physical environments." (page 68)

Each of these pioneering theorists are suggesting then, that social work practice must include at least two dimensions: (1) the direct treatment of patients and their families by the provision of counseling, referral and related services; and (2) treating the context of patient care, the organization and community as client systems. In other words, skilled social work interventions must be directed at the environments in which patient care occurs. The behaviors of hospital staff and systems as well as community agency personnel must be optimized and targeted for intervention when they are not functional. This framework has guided our practice at Huntington for years, elaborating on our initial blend of systems and crisis theory.

Direct Services

The theoretical framework has many implications for line staff and social work directors. The center of the diagram (Figure 1) is at the heart of things—the direct provision of clinical counseling, information and referral, discharge planning, education and other supportive and needed services for patients and their families. This is our primary mission.

Collaboration

That mission is then supported by a range of other key interventions that target the surrounding circles. These interventions are directed to the context in which patients and their families receive care in order to maximize that care, treating what Coulton calls "fit" and Germain refers to as "interface." The first such interface refers to the interdisciplinary nature of health care, i.e., the other caregivers who participate in patient care. A key social work role in health traditionally has included a range of education, advocacy, personal support and consultative activities with other professionals engaged in delivering care directly to patients. It is also important to work with other key hospital staff groups that have a direct impact on the patient, such as volunteers and housekeeping staff. We assumed this approach, interpreting these functions as basic to our mission from the inception of assuming the task of building a social work program. Fortunately, we found enough interest in the ideas to give us opportunities to demonstrate these concepts. As staff groups found us a helpful new resource, sanction for this role grew without serious resistance or opposition. It was a needed set of services and supports.

Hospital Systems

The next interface concerns working with the design of the broader hospital institution itself. The aim is to develop a hospital context that makes minimum damaging interventions with patients and is designed to promote optimum patient care. In this arena, systems social work practice entails the identification of hospital problem areas and active involvement in the development of new policies and institutional practices to address these concerns. Priority areas include the development of positive, constructive and non-damaging admissions procedures; ways of avoiding harrassment or other unnecessarily distressing behavior in the collection of payments; and ways of assuring access to the hospital through close involvement in the financial admissions requirements and types of insurances accepted. Participation in key hospital committees is also essential. Again, by assuming and identifying this role as within our scope and proving helpful in it, we gained acceptance and sanction for these facets of social work practice.

Hospital—Community Systems

The next circle portrays the interaction of the hospital patient care system with connecting agency care systems, be they convalescent hospitals, board and care facilities, shelters, child abuse protective services, law enforcement systems or others. The hospital interacts with and refers patients to a myriad of complex service-rendering systems with varying purposes. The obligation is to assure that our linkage with those systems is sound and constructive, and that it serves the needs of patients while respecting their right to privacy and confidentiality. The social work department has an obligation to assure that the systems to which it refers patients are responsive and provide appropriate and reasonable quality care and/or services. Participation at policy-making levels in these community organizations helps assure an informal power base which allows the social work department to generate high quality and timely results for patients when needed. It also facilitates efforts to make needed changes in the service delivery system design of these agencies where that is appropriate, based on feedback from referred patients. This has always been a formal aspect of professional practice in our department.

Developing, helping lead or coordinate, and participating in organized agency networking is also a vital area of practice. Networking helps assure coordinated care when multiple agencies are involved. It also improves agency practice through a timely mechanism for receiving feedback about the impact of your agency practice on clients and on receiving agencies. These staff activities not only improve the broader patient care system, they also lend balance to the clinicians' assignments, helping morale and staff development.

Research, Education, Social Policy

Finally, in the outer circle, involvement in research, professional and community education, and the development of broad social policy and legislation are vital activities. Research should occur at all levels of social work practice in order to provide objective feedback which assures that our interventions are in constructive, appropriate directions. Professional education is a critical activity, which, as it builds future professionals, applies research findings and disseminates practice wisdom, also improves social work practice in the setting and through the professional community.

Community education efforts are designed to empower clients and reduce the need for services through a preventive orientation. And finally, addressing social policy and legislation is a high form of advocacy. This is especially evident in the current environment of health care. Clearly, the social work perspective is a vital one in the redesign of the structure and financing mechanisms for the delivery of health services in the nation. Failure to translate experience at the bedside, in outpatient services and in the community into their broadest policy and legislative implications leaves us reacting to external changes rather than shaping the system itself.

Philosophically, social work administration is a form of social work practice dedicated to these same purposes. This theoretical framework guides both clinical and administrative practice in the health setting. The purpose of social work administration in health settings is to enable social work practice to occur with patients and their families, with staff, and with the institution itself. In fact, the social work department and the hospital as the host agency are the primary clients of the social work leader.

The basic responsibilities of the social work administrator as reported in the literature (Patti, 1983) are: Clarification of departmental purpose, and successful negotiation for financial resources, space and material supports. Recruitment, selection, deployment and retention of staff are priorities as well.

THE CHANGE PROCESS

Hospital and Department Missions Linked

Our effort to develop social work services at Huntington Memorial Hospital were initiated by the 1972 JCAH survey which urged that the hospital create a department that assured the availability of services to meet the psychological and social needs of all patients. The hospital responded with a positive view of this charge. It had grown dramatically from a medium sized hospital to a large regional medical center. Its managers were motivated to retain its tradition of highly personalized excellent care and to understand that this would be difficult in a larger institution. They viewed social work as an additional resource responsible for attending to the individualized needs of patients as well as for monitoring the design of hospital systems and services for their impact on maintaining warm and personalized care. Thus, our very birth as a department was rooted in a clear articulation of how we might address the needs of the hospital itself. This was a healthy position which we have retained throughout our existence. Viewing the hospital as a client and starting where the client was, we began with a positive acceptance of the status quo, which was that most physicians and other disciplines had not experienced the need for social work, had no clear idea of what social work should be and felt no particular interest in it. Beginning with comfort that we would have to work hard to develop understanding of social work and ability to use social work services appropriately put us in a positive and collaborative relationship with our many partners throughout the institution.

Staff as Pivotal Resources

In addition, we began with a positive view of change and operated from the belief that staff are our most essential resource. Therefore we wanted to build a system that was good for the social work staff as well as for the patients they cared for. We believed that staff who develop and who enjoy their jobs can provide the best care possible. And so we intentionally sought to design a system to support positive career development and satisfying professional experiences for line staff. We wanted strong staff who could enjoy taking hold of the opportunity to develop a service from scratch. This was a staff that was interested in making change and in helping to shape the direction of that change.

Evolutionary Pace of Change

Despite our recent growth spurt, gradual evolutionary change in manageable steps has been a way of life in this department. We are convinced that a slow pace of change allows for the maintenance of quality and the development of depth, and avoids the development of power struggles or creation of threats to others in the system. We are committed to an idiosyncratic and individually directed change process that seeks to match the talents and interests of individual staff members with emerging patient needs and available program opportunities in the system. Our premise was and is that there is limitless need and limited resources; and that the most efficient approach to program development and provision of high quality services is to follow a path of administratively enabling individual staff members to develop needed programs which interest them and which they wish to build. To the extent possible, control and direction of these programs remains in the hands of the prime mover staff member who initiated them. We have developed a program that provides social work services where they are wanted; and we continuously adapt and redesign these programs and services in light of patient input and staff comment. This approach has allowed us to build strong programs in areas where they were desired, which, in turn, gave us the opportunity to demonstrate to other areas the value of emerging social work services in the system. We developed strong interdisciplinary alliances and advocates; these frequently helped us expand staff during difficult times with advocacy on the part of our specialty clinical hosts within the hospital. This approach builds pride and a sense of ownership on the part of the staff and continues to push them to learn new skills and solve new problems.

Equally important, it is a patient centered model. For example, the first additional staff person employed in the department expanded her commitment to the quality of life for older patients to include interest in oncology services. Out of these concerns developed strong supportive counseling services, a sensitive, high quality approach to placement decision counseling, and active advocacy to assure return home whenever possible. As these services elaborated, advocacy for the development of a hospital oncology ward served as a foundation for physician leadership in this area and ultimately inspired the development of a home care Hospice in our community.

Major department developments were the results of slow growth based on persistent attention to understanding the needs of patients we were seeing and the availability of community services. This evolutionary collaborative process resulted in steady cumulative growth, with small accruals of staff, often quarter and half FTEs. Wherever possible we have introduced change naturally and imperceptibly. Early innovations occurred around the development of new hospital programs including neonatal intensive care, pediatric cardiology, rehabilitation care, cardiac rehabilitation and oncology. Building social work into these new programs was easier than adding social work to pre-existing programs. And it allowed us to establish a definition of social work based on the strongest specialty program models from other hospitals.

Key to this evolutionary model is a "behavior modification view of program development." We believe that the social work department's reputation is based on the strength and quality of the last observed performance. Moving initially from a "one down" and mildly sanctioned posture, we are committed to swift and excellent clinical responses to referrals. There is a credo that staff never say "no," but rather assist people in determining how to obtain an appropriate hospital staff response to an identified need. In addition, feedback to a referral source is rapid and thorough in order to share ownership of the clinical outcome achieved by social work. Twenty-four hour on-call for emergencies and consultation helped build our credibility.

We move swiftly and undefensively to respond to criticisms of services, evincing interest and eagerness to solve problems identified. Finally, high quality interpersonal relationships with physicians, nurses and members of other disciplines are vital to building a base from which effective communication of our social work services and concepts can be conveyed. Walking slowly, spending time with others in conversation about patients and staff needs, asking the advice of other disciplines, and high quality charting have been key approaches, although these are increasingly threatened by the growing stress in today's hospital care systems.

Finally, respect for staff is consciously equal to the regard in which we hold our clients. Respect for clients is our highest standard and seemed the appropriate level of regard in which to hold all human beings in the system. The needs of staff are considered as important as the needs of clients. This approach has helped us to build a highly reciprocal system designed to work for all affected by it, one that is responsive to requests for service and input for needed change.

Articulation of social work services and concepts has been based on generalizing to a description of services after an opportunity to demonstrate them had become available. We were careful not to offer general concepts without practical illustrations and cautious not to make promises that could not be kept. Ultimately our best sales program was to deliver high quality clinical services based on the premise that appropriate utilization of social work services would best emerge from seeing them first and then hearing our professional description of what had been observed to elaborate the understanding. These strategies served to promote acceptance of social work services and their integration in the clinical practice arena.

Building Management Credibility

The opportunity to demonstrate social work services at the administrative level through assisting relatives and friends of administrators was analogous. But here, in addition to clinical credibility, the development of managerial credibility was the cornerstone of the change process. Building the understanding and use of social work services and developing collegial advocates for increased social work resources could only succeed by working consistently to cut through the stereotypes about social work as a discipline; and to establish the social work department head as an effective and contributing member of the hospital's management team.

Several principles guided our practice in this arena. First, I worked hard to assure that no surprises came to administrators responsible for the social work department. Problems, complaints or conflicts were immediately brought to their attention so that they came from us rather than an outside source. Suggestions for changes in the hospital or the social work system were developed carefully, based on a preceding period in which anecdotal information was offered to identify and establish agreement about existence of a problem that needed solving. Careful collaboration and consensus building efforts resulted in bringing forward modest suggestions for change; we made sure to err conservatively on the side of complete accuracy rather than risk our reputation for sound administrative judgment. Critical, too, is an alert, continuing attention to the hospital's changing needs over time, its shifting values and budgetary concerns carefully tracked and identified. Needed development of social work services and programs is articulated clearly in terms of how they address the primary needs of the hospital and the administrator's natural concern for its fiscal and clinical strength and excellence. Development of a highly reciprocal model of mutual benefit to client, hospital staff and the integrity of social work design is an abiding principle that heightens a slow, steady growth. The establishment of the Senior Care Network was based on this same concern for helping maintain a strong hospital through our own development.

Achieving Consensus Through Collaboration

The cutting edge of departmental excellence occurs in the implementation of the leadership role. A cornerstone of effective leadership is the development of consensus building skills to mobilize existing human resources on behalf of a common goal. True power rests on the ability to build consensus about shared values and goals and to build agreement and methods for achieving them. The creation of a shared vision of a desirable future is a vital component of administrative leadership within the social work department and the hospital. Building networks of interdisciplinary and interagency commitment to needed systems modifications is the mark of an effective changemaker. Harkening back to Figure 1, the social work administrator has an obligation to treat the interface between the client/family and the systems with which they interface. The clinician's effort focuses on treating the client, identifying barriers to optimum interactions with external environments and addressing those barriers. The administrative task is to respond to the social work clinician's identification of (1) general problems in hospital operations, (2) policies, problems in the functioning of external community agencies and (3) problems resulting from impact of legislation and broad social policy.

For example, the hospital needs state-of-the-art, high quality clinical programs that are innovative, of interest to the community and satisfying to the medical staff and patients. The hospital also needs to remain economically viable. Social work wants to provide high quality social work services the patient needs and can utilize. A clinical/administrative program marriage was created when it was discerned that patients in the cardiac rehabilitation program had significant problems managing stress and yet were not amenable to traditional counseling and educational techniques. The social work department was able to develop a biofeedback/stress management training program on a fee-for-service basis (utilizing the hospital's charitable funds where patients were unable to pay). This enhanced clinical services by creating a new service that had high publicity value for the hospital and developing it into a self supporting program with potential revenue producing capability. This program development effort was a distinct partnership between client, clinician and administrator. Clearly one cannot do without the other.

With the Community

The measure of the wisdom and effectiveness of any given institutional or societal social policy or practice is its impact on the individual. The administrator must ask: does this approach work effectively on behalf of human beings and human services? This knowledge can only be garnered at the clinical level, from hearing the tales of individual and family experiences and seeing the fruits of agency and community systems on their lives. For this reason administrators cannot effectively lead policy-making efforts without a client-centered information base to point the way. Social work clinicians, on the other hand, while active advocates and policy makers in their interface with hospital and community systems, often cannot lend the time to focus interventions at the macro level. These two staff levels need to operate hand in hand, marching toward common objectives in differential ways. A system that effectively addresses system problems helps maintain clinician optimism.

The director draws from the collective clinical experience to inspire macro-interventions to frame social policy and to build an optimum network of linked community caregiving systems. In our theoretical framework, hospital-based social work administrative practice also requires addressing the multiple community interfaces in the continuum of care. The patient passes through many caregiving systems both internally and in the community. Optimum patient care, especially of vulnerable populations, rests on building effective networks of care for shared patients. For administrative success in this circle, close linkages with law enforcement, legal systems, residential and other community care and financing systems are essential. Otherwise these systems work at odds rather than in concert and dilute the impact of each other's efforts to improve patients' lives. Interagency networks for child abuse and rape treatment are good examples. This model of practice is essential for care of the elderly and the disabled as well. The social work director sets an expectation and creates a work standard that includes this clinical posture. Active involvement of hospital social work staff in community planning for human services is critical in building an optimum, comprehensive approach to client needs. It also is valuable in varying the workload of line staff and building in a broader perspective and a climate for excellence.

The sanction for the concept that all professional social work staff will participate in community-based practice was garnered by utilizing the strategy of gradual, incremental and almost imperceptible change. Our approach utilized making changes at an informal level to develop precedent and then formalizing them after practice has been accepted. In the instance of community involvement, we began initially with the director requesting the opportunity to accept an invitation to serve on a local community board. That board led to committee assignments. Acquaintances made led to the opportunity to network with other key agencies serving common groups of clients. Once the request to legitimate participation in community activities was approved on a one-time basis, we were able to elaborate that for the director and other staff with only modest reporting. When this sphere of activity expanded to a major level of activity, a standard was set by administration. It was agreed that as long as services to patients remained available immediately and at a high level of quality, the department could maintain its policy of asking staff to participate in a minimum of one outside community agency activity at a time in order to prevent burnout, maintain perspective and enhance our policy-making and advocacy capabilities. This was written into job descriptions, built into our pre-employment interviewing and new employee orientation. This supports our hypothesis that the definition of the social work department is determined largely by the activities the department elects to engage in. It is difficult to receive a formal sanction without a base of experience. It is fairly simple to receive a formal sanction for an activity that has become the status quo.

With Hospital Staff and Administrators

Collaboration/networking is crucial at another level as well. Building resources and programs for hospital social work cannot occur in isolation. Both the clinical service design and the resource allocation process occur with the close involvement and essential support of a range of colleagues. Here internal networking in the hospital system is the primary focus. This occurs at all levels of departmental leadership but is the primary responsibility of the administrative leader. The role definition, sanctions for social work services and approvals of budget for staff and material resources must have the active support and advocacy of a host of persons. Building this agreement comes through interaction and conjoint planning.

The strength of a social work budget request is enhanced if the chief physician of a service, several hospital administrators affected by the decision but not responsible for the budgeting question and/or nursing management take the lead in seeking increased services, new directions and improved financial and material resources. Whether this takes the form of complaints that social work services are inadequate to achieve a desired outcome or that new resources are needed to move the hospital care system to a higher level of excellence, the outside intervention is crucial to lending credibility to the request. Collaborative practice must pervade the social work system and all its interfaces with colleagues in the hospital organization. It is insufficient to have excellent relationships at the top if there are not excellent relationships throughout all levels of social work and colleague interaction.

There is a posture implicit in collaborative practice, a tone which must be set by the social work administrative leadership team. This is a posture familiar to the clinician, that of acceptance: starting where the other person is. We do this automatically with the client. It is central to our training. Critical to effective social work practice in a host setting is bringing this dynamic to the collegial framework. There can be no double standard here. The client cannot receive better treatment than the colleague or the administrator or board member. A rose is a rose . . . a person is a person is a person. This kind of respect or mutuality, drawing on the clinical listening skills and the capacity for empathy, is crucial to true collaboration at all levels, including staff of the social work department.

Collaborative practice brings together two or more disparate perspectives and enriches the final outcome through the interaction and synergy of these perspectives. It is not the dominance of one profession or one person over another. It is the democratic process at its best, real respect for difference and what it has to offer us. This valuing of pluralism, internally and in relationships with all who interface with a social work department, is based on mutuality. It is important, also, in the relationships within the department. Slippage in respect and candor about differences in the internal collegial system results in major disruptions and the investment of significant emotional energy in staff issues at the expense of patient care. Reciprocity is the key term here. There are no long term winners when there are losers in the conjoint and shared planning process which develops social work services to serve a hospital and community system.

Reciprocity is also essential in the social work director's interface with hospital administration. The concept of institutional maintenance and reciprocity in achieving the social work mission in a manner supportive to the hospital mission is germane. In marketing social work programs to the hospital, the method for describing the value of clinical social work services must highlight their benefits for institutional maintenance. In addition to meeting the needs of patients and their families the social work director must identify the contributions of social work to the financial viability of the hospital. For example, social work services reduce the risk of malpractice suits as well as the length of time required to collect payment for patient care. They increase the stability and quality of the patient care staff through EAP services. The social worker provides clinical services because of the primary professional values that guide practice. The hospital utilizes and pays for clinical social work services for patients and staff at an optimum level when they also understand the additional secondary effects just described. For example, the clinical social work staff are dedicated to the development of an optimum set of services to care for the elderly. While the hospital shares this goal, it must consider additional factors when allocating major resources for new programs. For instance, being a leader in clinical quality and establishing new approaches to this population may result in an enhanced reputation, leading to a significant census/volume increase, a critical financial survival issue for the host institution. Development of a coordinated care program may be valued as an experience base for managing at-risk, capitated care contracts.

In summary then, the capacity of the social work administrator to articulate institutional (hospital) benefit from particular direct social work services programs is a key to success in garnering strong, reliable sanction and funding for services. Since the provision of the resources necessary for the effective delivery of social work services is the first purpose of the social work administrator, these perspectives and capabilities are central to success in building consensus with the host setting.

With Social Work Staff

In this context, the heart of its internal administrative leadership lies in conceptualizing, articulating and sustaining a vision of a new future that the department works to build. This vision defines a mission that motivates staff to elevate their practice to a level of outstanding performance. It spurs clinical excellence in interaction with patients and their families. It inspires the staff to establish and maintain superb relationships with colleagues in the hospital's care-giving teams in the face of daily stresses. It is crucial to assure effective, ongoing integration of social work in health care, with proper utilization and appropriate referrals. It also contributes to staff willingness to "go the extra mile," to rise to difficult professional circumstances effectively. It helps encourage staff to move important incidents observed in individual interactions in the hospital to the policy making process. As a department grows in size, this view must be shared and directly imparted by the supervisors.

A variety of methods are utilized to articulate the collaboratively developed vision of the mission of the social work department. The pre-employment screening process is a critical structure for building appropriate expectations about the nature of practice in the setting and for identifying and selecting clinicians whose interests and skills are compatible with that approach. This base line information is reinforced throughout the orientation of new staff. In addition, we have developed a formal departmental orientation which articulates this vision of social work practice. A thorough review of the department's history and its values also serve as a basis to convey the impact that individual staff members can have in the growth of the department through building programs around their emerging interests and talents in the care of patients. The department's written materials, especially its policy and procedure manual, reflect a consistency with this vision. Staff must learn to articulate this view themselves in order to interpret consistently the role and function of the department on a daily basis in their interface with colleagues throughout the medical center.

In our department adding the graduate student clinical training program created new avenues for articulating and teaching these concepts. Opportunities to lecture at the local graduate school of social work also helped fine-tune the articulation of these concepts and create a clear understanding in the community of this direction and definition of social work practice in health. These multiple strategies worked together to help build a consensus which is sustained best by maintaining practice standards which actually reflect the clinical philosophy described.

Administrative practice, a major statement of administrative values and concerns, is reflected in the nature of problems identified and addressed and the methods used for these interventions. Social work administration intervenes with explicit concern in ways which assure appropriate supports for high quality social work practice, support staff testing new concepts without fear of criticism and remove administrative barriers to the development of pilot projects which test emerging practice ideas.

This perspective of a broader vision supports open exploration of how things can and should be gives clinicians the hope and the energy required to invest themselves in changing the environment with which they interact. The best clinical work, strong interfaces with the hospital clinical and administrative systems and energetic advocacy to build constructive hospital and community agency policies are undergirded by administrative values, behaviors and systems. These are needed to support the implementation of the consummate social work vision of patient-environment interaction by a stable and high morale staff. The leadership team must create expectations, approaches and rewards, in partnership with the staff, that free staff to build a collegial environment based on mutual respect and reciprocal support. This is essential so that critical human resources are not dissipated in internal conflicts. In the hospital setting, staff face daily stressors and difficult circumstances and they, themselves, need support and attention. The personnel of the social work department are its basic tool and its greatest resource. As an administrative team, we have given conscious attention to internal team building in order to establish an atmosphere in which there is the safety to communicate directly enough to resolve the inevitable and inherent internal conflicts as well as to risk error in the interest of seeking innovation.

In addition, it is critical for leaders to sustain an intensive communication and problem solving effort aimed at building positive collegial support systems, healthy conflict resolution and effective management of differences within the department. This, too, requires reiteration from pre-employment interviews through orientation and ongoing dialogue via existing staff structures including staff meetings, team meetings and our cross team quarterly meetings known fondly as "fireside chats."

THE SOCIAL WORK ADMINISTRATOR AS LEADER

I believe that central to the social work administrator's role as leader is building an optimum environment in which excellent work can occur. Critical to the success of this effort is the ability to build an environment based on caring professional commitment, hope, persistence, and fairness. These critical elements are essential to creating a work environment in which people can put forth their best without being distracted into concerns about repair of the immediate environment.

The leader's optimism sets the posture of the department relative to its host setting. If the leader believes that things cannot be changed, that difficult challenges cannot be mastered constructively or that the influence of social work cannot be brought to bear upon the institution in the significant ways needed to optimize health care, social work staff will either follow in kind or will feel frustrated by the lack of strong top level advocacy.

Staff generally assume that the social work administrator has relatively complete information and therefore that his/her assessment of circumstances is correct. Crises will come, especially in these times of great change. In essence, the social work administrative leader sets the tone for addressing crises within the department and within the institution. Individuals will expend their energy in striving for high level solutions when they have permission/sanction for this work, when they are helped to develop and articulate a vision of what is possible, and when they are convinced that progress is possible. Since positive change rarely occurs from a single intervention, and since people so easily give up hope that the status quo can be changed, an inherent part of the leadership role is to interpret the significance of continuing efforts, to interpret the impact of efforts made along the way to illustrate that gradual change is occurring, and to encourage continuing advocacy efforts.

For example, in our hospital the need for specialty services for children in Pediatrics were identified. It was determined that child development specialist staff needed to be brought on board to establish a play room and a therapeutic play program to help reduce the trauma of illness and hospitalization and help children better manage their concerns and feelings about hospital experiences. This need was identified early in our history and our ability to introduce a new concept of this sort was challenged. The proposal was presented over a two or three year period both in formal and informal budgeting efforts. Finally we were successful in being authorized to hire a half-time child development specialist to develop the new program which has subsequently evolved into a highly valued and physician supported program which is instrumental in enhancing the quality of staff, patient and family life in the pediatrics units. Persistence for the development of this and other programs, sustaining the effort in the face of a significant number of reversals and disappointments and continuously finding new approaches and new ways to articulate, identify and address solutions to the problem were essential.

In fact, the capacity to persist in a task is an attribute critical to success in program building. Here there are several important considerations.

First, most important goals do take continuing and persistent interventions over a period of time, much like the long-term therapeutic process. Important changes do not occur easily or as a result of single interventions. Incremental change is difficult to measure and document. Fear of failure complicates this effort and is compounded by the tendency to believe that the efforts of a single person can not make a major difference in systems change or systems interactions. And yet the excellent setting is characterized by its distinctive ability to sustain endeavors to produce fine outcomes. Setting this tone, sustaining this effort and inspiring the direction for unified effort is a critical leadership function.

Perhaps even more crucial than the likelihood of success is the emotional and symbolic significance of unceasing efforts. Many staff systems, almost without one's noticing it, seem to give up hope about their long-range impact on the environment where patients and staff interface. Can things really be improved? What kind of change is possible? Is it worth continuing to try? Does what I do really make a difference? While answering these in the affirmative leads to potential excellence, answering them in the negative puts a professional department at risk. Giving up is the first step to despair, a form of professional depression. Maintaining hope and optimism sufficient to persistent pursuit of departmental goals is central to organizational health.

Administrative credibility inside the department is also predicated upon a perception of caring leaders who value "fairness." This is a complex, multi-faceted phenomenon reflecting the establishment of a belief that management can be "trusted" to respect the needs and capabilities of staff and to create an environment with organizational reciprocity. Internal trust among the staff, both vertically and horizontally, is essential to a balanced operation with a productive internal equilibrium. As growth occurs and promotional opportunities arise, "fairness" credibility is essential.

Beyond a shared department goal, there must be a shared set of values, an agreed-upon philosophy of the work itself, the amount, the type, the approaches used. Standards must be widely shared and the work effort viewed as a shared product, owned by all, whose outcomes rest on the efforts of each individual. As the department has matured, the increasing use of committees has helped create forums for internal collaboration.

The administrator must view the department and its staff as an assigned "client." Organizational health is the objective. As in a clinical relationship, nothing can proceed well until trust is established. Given the infusion of the authority and power differential inherent in the "boss-staff" relationship, a variety of special efforts are usually necessary to assure a balanced, healthy internal department environment.

There is a constellation of attributes that can help free staff to address their full energies to patient care rather than struggles with internal departmental issues. One such attribute is the maintenance of clinical and staff interaction standards. Setting clear expectations at the time of employment is important. Clarifying them at the inevitable junctures when teams divide internally is essential. Team building behaviors, demonstrating mutual respect with colleagues, handling conflicts directly, tolerating differences, these are conditions of employment. The administrator must be seen as both supportive and demanding. Rules, policies, assignments must have demonstrated fairness. There must also be enough safety and margin of error to make it safe to try new approaches, to innovate and to share untested ideas and concepts.

Within this context, staff members work best in a system that wants and acknowledges their best effort. This must come from the leadership in the form of high expectations combined with respect for and acknowledgement of achievement. When these standards are being undermined by poor staff performance, productive staff need to see administrative corrective action. This "proves" the high standards are valued. A healthy system rests on clear and direct feedback designed to assure timely praise *and* correction in an observably fair and consistent manner. Excellence, one's best effort, is predicated on the presumption that it will make a difference, that it will be known, rewarded and acknowledged. Maintaining these values in an environment that supports sustained good work is a critical leadership task. Stopping poor work and handling negative attitudes quickly, calmly and with fair due process is essential in this area of administrative practice.

The other critical element is fair representation and maintenance of hope about the ongoing negotiation for policies and resources for the department. The administrator serves as the voice of the department, seeking resources needed to maintain excellent effort at the service level. It is essential to believe that the manager/leader is representing staff's and clients' needs effectively. It is vital for staff to know that their administrator advocates for the improvement of hospital policies and practices to enhance patient care. One can live with a problem if one is certain that all possible is being done to solve it. If not, a form of apathy/despair/depression sets in and it becomes difficult to perform optimal work.

The same is true with shortfalls in resource allocation. A staff shortage can be tolerated with good morale if hope exists that solutions will be found. This hope relies on the administrator holding and demonstrating an optimistic and persistent posture in seeking resources. It is not the outcomes alone that have impact but the interpretation of the effort, the rationale for a decision and the capacity to engage staff in ongoing efforts in the face of adversity. If the leader gives up or despairs of better times, the staff may well follow suit. If, instead, the director views a "defeat" as one outcome in a continuing series of negotiations, the staff have a much better chance of maintaining good morale and sustained good work. Wherever possible, we encourage staff involvement in the efforts of department and patient advocacy in order to share ownership of the department and avoid a sense of helplessness. These efforts to build shared goals and common values, to maintain good work and constructive collegial interaction, to engage staff in problem-solving, to maintain hope and persistence until an acceptable outcome occurs, are key in building internal reciprocity and equilibrium.

ADVANCING THE STATUS OF THE PROFESSION

Developing a system with vision, perspective and persistence is especially vital to social work administration because social work tends to experience a distinct form of prejudice in a majority of hospital settings. We don't have an "ism" for it, like racism or sexism, but a comparable form of stereotyping and prejudice affects social work departments in most hospitals. It is important to conceptualize this phenomenon since it is a primary dynamic with which social work administrators and staff work on a daily basis.

In broad terms, the social work department is often seen by both administrators and staff of other disciplines through a screen of misconceptions and assumptions. It is assumed that social workers are bleeding hearts, hand-holders, not cost-conscious and so on. They are not viewed as a clinically essential element of the patient care system. Their expertise as mental health practitioners is often denied or unknown. As our department grew in our early years, we faced these perceptions directly. They persist as new staff who join the hospital need orientation to our social work services system.

This prejudice is a culturally-based phenomenon which requires an analysis of each hospital area and staff group to assess where medical staff, administrators and other colleagues lie on its continuum and what inaccurate preconceptions they may carry about social work. This is a diagnostic formulation that sets the focus for our collegial interventions. A hospital is not clinically complete without a strong social work component. The task is to assist members of the patient care teams and administration to gradually develop an accurate understanding of our discipline. It is helpful to conceptualize this as a continuum of hospital receptivity to social work, a normal spectrum of acceptance. Any specific hospital or unit will fall somewhere on the continuum. The social work department can start at that point and work for forward movement. This point of view removes the insult and discomfort from the syndrome. Looking back at our department's early development, we developed the following conceptual framework.

Levels of Acceptance

Five levels of acceptance were identified to reflect five departmental developmental stages. Each stage of receptivity has select diagnostic indicators which can be utilized to see where a particular department and hospital falls on this spectrum of hospital acceptance of social work services.

An analogy for the early stages of acceptance is that of "transplant": when a social work department is first introduced to a medical care system, we can recognize a phenomenon akin to organ transplant. A foreign object (social work) is introduced to an intact system which has struck a balance internally in relation to its external environment with which it is relatively satisfied. For example, a visit from the Joint Commission is due and the hospital believes it must have some form of social work. It introduces the "foreign object" of social work to the system and a whole series of potential rejection problems arise. Resistances can be anticipated. There is an integration problem. The initial introduction or expansion of social work to a hospital system is much like an affirmative action hire. The department is usually subjected to stereotypical perceptions on the part of other members of the hospital system. Common terms heard at this point are that social workers are bleeding hearts, handholders, software, too expensive, unessential, and so on. These, as noted, are not accurate perceptions of social work, but rather are common, stereotypical thinking on the part of medical personnel and hospital administrators. Still social work is a required service. And from an affirmative action point of view, even though it may be with discomfort, the hospital is required to have at least token social work programming. This then is the *tokenism stage* of the five levels of acceptance.

In this stage it is common in many hospitals to utilize a part-time consultant, to appoint an inappropriate designee, or perhaps to hire a single social worker as Huntington hired me. In such a circumstance there are few friendly faces available to the "affirmative action hire." The overall tone is commonly one of reluctance, ambivalence, distant neutrality, and misperception of the service. Most people believe that social work should be a small service for the poor, providing charitable assistance, serving Medicaid patients and doing a range of other simple concrete tasks delegated by other members of the medical care team. Many hospitals remain in this first stage for years: social work has weak standing as a professional discipline and there is no broad conceptualization of the discipline's role. Obviously, strategies at this time are educational and trust-building. No radical changes can occur in such a climate. This is simply a time to form relationships and begin the very first steps in building a base of support within the system. This was our experience at Huntington. We built relationships deliberately and carefully and sought opportunities to demonstrate the clinical contribution of social work. After consistent, slow, steady trust-building efforts, the social work department may move from tokenism and the affirmative-action-hire position to the second stage of acceptance, which we call *conditional acceptance.*

In this stage there is a reluctant decline in animosity: "you're not quite as bad as we thought," others seem to be saying. We were glad when fewer hospital staff poked fun at us or refused to trust that we had value. Here is the beginning of individualizing, some staff are beginning to develop trusting relationships with social workers. Some begin to refer cases and begin to see social work practice in action. Other staff will continue to watch with less active resistance, but still certain that social work is unnecessary in health care. If all goes well, some limited and cautious notice begins to be taken of the value of social work services. More referrals begin to come in, some personal respect develops, which forms a basis for professional respect and acceptance. In our case the chief physician and head nurse in the Emergency Department developed an interest in our work and helped us begin to grow.

The third stage is the *exception syndrome.* Here the particular social worker and/or social work department are viewed positively, but the broad discipline of social work is viewed negatively. You are likely to hear new comments in the hallway. Members of the medical staff, nursing, and possibly administration begin to make remarks like, "we still hate social work, but we do like you." This is definitely an improvement over the first stage, but obviously a very limited level of acceptance and understanding of the appropriate social work role within the hospital system. We experienced this and found it an important risk point. Conceptualizing it helps us to not "fall for it," as the implicit personal aggrandisement can be seductive.

As the fourth stage approaches, you begin to hear new conversations and hallway comments that evidence some movement towards the broader acceptance of social work as a professional service and discipline, rather than only approving of an individual staff member as an exception to the rule. More resources begin to be allocated, a result of growing administrative trust that the social work department makes sense and has some kind of a valid role to play with the institution. And the hallway comments begin to sound something like "I don't know what we did before we had you; what did we do before social work was here?" There is recognition of a valuable contribution that other disciplines have come to rely and depend upon. When we began, we had predicted that moving to what we now call the fourth level of acceptance, a normative expectation, would be a ten year plan. We joked about how having this long range perspective assisted us in developing the patience and acceptance we needed to comfortably and persistently continue to interact in a manner designed to promote further understanding and appropriate utilization of social work services throughout the medical center in the face of some pockets of persistent misconception. While progress was uneven throughout the hospital, it did, in fact require between eight and ten years to develop a reasonably accurate understanding of social work throughout the clinical and administrative areas of the hospital.

At this fourth level, *the normative expectation level,* the hospital has integrated social work as a full-fledged clinical team member, an essential organ in the hospital system. There is no need to give approval to the role of accepted disciplines. No one says, "I'm glad we have doctors," or "what would we do without the nurses" or, "what did we do before the nurses were here?" They are an assumed part of the system; this is the way things are and ought to be. When social work enters this level, the hallway conversations become one of complaint if social work does not maintain its appropriate service level.

Here the glory of being an exception and a pleasant surprise ends. Having won respect, the task now is to keep it and build on it. Ironically, indicators of positive regard are now often negative. Complaints come from failure to meet the now high expectations of the department. Other staff become concerned if social work is absent or not there fast or effectively enough. The department now is viewed as an essential service, and like X-ray, expected to be and remain available. In this context, complaints can be a compliment as they indicate a high expectation and a reliance by another discipline on social work input. Such concerns should be welcomed and worked with as opportunities to continue to support the view of other caregivers and administrators in the system that the social worker is indeed essential and must be available in a timely and competent way. Social work is now more automatically or easily built into new programs.

It has proven very useful for the social work staff at Huntington Memorial to conceptualize these stages of assimilation and acceptance, especially this last stage. This allows us to retain a healthy perspective about negative input about our services and to continue to view candid, negative feedback as a tribute to people's belief that we desire to give optimum services and will correct problems based on their input. It remains important to reinforce this view.

The fifth stage is emerging now for us and is seen in the focus of this book. It may be called the stage of *assimilation into the upper power structure of the hospital.* This is a stage where the social work director is promoted to take responsibility for more than the social work department. This can be a strong and practical acknowledgement of the social work department's value to the total institution, an important measure of impact. It may even reflect a shift in conscious institutional values, as our "soft" contributions are viewed as clinically vital, economically valuable and cost-effective. Ideally, the promotion of the director takes social work up with it as an acknowledgement both of the strengths of the social work director and the professional perspective for health planning that social work training and practice provide. There is a risk of another form of the exception syndrome at this stage of assimilation. Leaving social work behind at this juncture strips the profession of its strongest leaders and deprives the director of the department's essential, key data base. Integration of social work and the director's promotion is crucial for both.

CONCLUSION

The health care system is undergoing radical redesign, some of it clear and some not so clearly understood. This time of rapid change represents a time of risk that many strengths will be damaged. It also offers a unique opportunity for reform, for meaningfully addressing key problems in the traditional health care system.

Regardless of the stage of development of the social work department in a given hospital, we have been convinced by our experience at Huntington Memorial Hospital that reciprocity, collaboration, consensus building and shared ownership of the social work department by all levels of social work staff as well as key outside allies is critical to its success. A free-standing, talented leader would not provide sufficient strength to achieve the outcomes discussed in this chapter. Strong clinical social work staff are the most essential resource a department has. Developing a strong outside reputation is vital as a recruitment tool. A thoughtful and well developed screening and selection process is crucial to developing the kind of fit that will build a positive, constructive social work team. Maintaining strong, internal communication systems to assure proper flow of information between clinical and administrative systems is the cornerstone of sound planning and program development. Assisting staff in developing and maintaining appropriate support systems and methods for managing differences cannot long be neglected without quickly depleting a positive and practice-enhancing collegial community. Mutual loyalty among social work administrators and between social work line staff is essential; these two strong systems must then be linked into a cohesive whole dedicated to bringing their differential talents and perspectives to the building of an optimum health care system with significant social work influence at the heart of its decision-making process and clinical designs.

A blend of strong, shared staff ownership of the system, hospital-wide collaboration and conscious building of services that are clearly seen as supporting the clinical and financial health of the hospital itself, must be coupled with a strong partnership with all key community partners including consumers, providers of services to specialty populations and other systems which have impact on patient care and community care processes. These guiding principles and the opportunity to participate in state and national education and policy development activities contributed to the development of social work and ultimately to its exciting new programs emerging as the Senior Care Network. Delivering social work services to patients at Huntington Memorial Hospital laid the base of understanding that enabled us to put forth ideas so well targeted that major funding emerged to assure their implementation.

The comprehensive, patient-centered view of the systems-design-oriented social work administrator has special value in this context, resulting in many promotions across this nation in recent years. Promotion is one method of infusing the social work perspective into health planning. Remaining a strong key manager in the more familiar role of social work department leader is equally crucial. The essential issue is assuring that our nation's health care system retain balance, treating the whole person while assuring full access and informed consent. Social work leadership skills and qualities are crucial at every level of that system.

REFERENCES

Coulton, Claudia J. "A Study of Person-Environment Fit Among the Chronically Ill," *Social Work in Health Care*, 5 (1) 1979, pp. 5–18.

Germain, Carel B. "An Ecological Perspective on Social Work in Health Care," *Social Work in Health Care*, 3 (1) 1977, pp. 67–77.

Patti, Rino J. *Social Welfare Administration*, Englewood Cliffs, N.J.: Prentice-Hall, 1983.

Pincus, Allen and Anne Minahan, *Social Work Practice: Model and Method*, Itasca, Ill: F.E. Peacock, 1973.

CHAPTER X

Alternatives and Options: The Transition from Social Work Director to Hospital Administrator

Patricia J. Volland, MSW, MBA

CURRENT POSITION AND RESPONSIBILITIES

I am the Senior Director for Patient Services at the Johns Hopkins Hospital.* My promotion occurred in January, 1982 when this senior management position was created as part of a hospitalwide reorganization whose major intent was to provide leadership for the development and maintenance of Patient Services to maximize the utilization of the Hospital's resources while at the same time, maintaining high quality patient care. My current operational responsibilities include: Admitting Office, Medical Records, Home Care Services, Social Work, and Patient Relations and Volunteer Services. As Senior Director for Patient Services, I am responsible for ensuring that these services provided by the above departments are provided to the patients' served by the decentralized clinical departments. These decentralized clinical departments include: Medicine, Surgery, Pediatrics, Psychiatry, Oncology, Neurosciences, Opthalmology, and Emergency Medicine. The focus of the patient services are the following:

1. Efficient and improved utilization of Hospital resources with

---

*Ms. Volland is now Vice President, Planning and Development, Deaton Hospital, Baltimore, MD.

resultant high occupancy in inpatient areas and improvement i
outpatient/inpatient interface.
2. Improvement in the quality of patient care services.
3. Support and enhancement of the services provided by the abov
   identified decentralized clinical departments, called Functiona
   Units.
4. Provision of needed longterm care services to Hospital patients.
5. Improvement in communications with patient care entry points t
   ensure better coordination and triaging of service to patients.
6. Improvement of the working relationships with the financia
   division of the Hospital to maximize revenues within the frame
   work of improved patient care services.

I also carry administrative responsibility for managing a nine millio
dollar budget associated with the House Staff who are engaged i
postdoctoral education at The Johns Hopkins University, School o
Medicine, and who provide primary patient care services to John
Hopkins Hospital patients. This assignment carries with it primar
responsibility for ensuring that patient care needs and educational goal
are effectively coordinated. I serve as administrative liaison to th
Womens's Board, a group dedicated to supporting the interest of th
Hospital through financial and community commitments. As Senio
Director, I am also the principle investigator for several grants associate
with the development and improvement of longterm and community car
services to the Hospital's patient population.

A major facet in this position is the opportunity to participate in the
development of Hospital policy and future planning. At this Hospital,
senior managers are encouraged to take on additional responsibilities and
projects with a look toward future program possibilities. Thus, there
are opportunities for planning and implementing special projects.
Examples of projects in which I have participated include: the development and direction of programs to reduce length of stay to ensure medical
and financial success under prospective pricing; designing, marketing,
and implementing a home health care program to reduce length of stay
and guarantee an expanding patient market; designing and implementing
a computerized system that produces a single clinical resume at the end
of an inpatient episode of care; creation and implementation of admissions policies that produce increased occupancy and additional revenue;
and organizing and managing an uncompensated care program designed
to reduce bad debts while insuring access to services for the uninsured
medically ill.

Our Hospital is well known for its decentralized management structure
(Heyssel et al., 1984). Each clinical department is a Functional Unit
responsible for revenues and expenses associated with providing patient

care services; the management of each Functional Unit is shared by a trio of managers including a physician chief, nursing director, and an administrator. Services and functions that remain centrally controlled, which includes the Patient Services Division, have an especially delicate challenge in this organization to ensure high quality services in the clinical structure. Those centrally provided services must meet the expectation of the Functional Units, and enhance the delivery of patient care services at the lowest possible cost.

This position of Senior Director for Patient Services was created at a time when the Hospital leadership anticipated marked changes in the health care delivery system. The President and Trustees were aware that competition would soon require higher levels of efficiency and began to focus on patient satisfaction issues. At that time, it was recognized that the Hospital needed to become more concerned about alternative delivery sites for patient care to ensure our market share, and ensure the opportunity to provide high quality services to our patient population at low cost sites. These particular issues convinced the Hospital leadership that a new organizational structure was needed as a foundation for becoming increasingly effective in a competitive health care environment.

SOCIAL WORK MANAGEMENT EXPERIENCE

What prepared me as Social Work Director to participate in the Hospital's decision to reorganize? Answering this question requires an assessment of the components associated with success as a Director of the Department of Social Work. Two integral components of this role are management skills and demonstrated leadership. Management abilities include the development and implementation of planning, fiscal management, policy generation, personnel and program evaluations as well as effective interpersonal skills. According to Drucker (1974), an expert in management science, management is defined as follows:

> Management is tasks. Management is a discipline. But management is also people. Every achievement of management is the achievement of a manager. Every failure is a failure of a manager. People manage, rather than "forces" or "facts." The vision, dedication, and integrity of managers determine whether there is management or mismanagement.

Since leadership is classified as the process of taking charge of certain events or situations and of encouraging participation, the successful manager is a person who utilizes leadership skills effectively, and attains respect of subordinates, peers, and superiors with sufficient expertise to exert authority and influence in getting the job done.

Within this context, the Social Work Director in a major teaching hospital has the primary responsibility to demonstrate the economic value of social work services within the institution. Why is this a crucial activity? At the time I assumed the position of Director of the Department of Social Work at the Hospital in 1973, it was evident that financial support for health care was in a transitional phase.

The Hospital leadership recognized this, and in order to ensure future service delivery opportunities they had already begun to focus on increased efficiency and effectiveness. In addition, one of the Hospital's major goals was to provide high quality patient care at the most reasonable cost. Therefore, it became essential to correlate social work practice with the financial viability of the Hospital. This was accomplished through the development of a comprehensive discharge planning program that ensured the patient's return to the community with adequate plans, and which minimized the non-paid days of care in the Hospital (administratively necessary days). In this program, social work services were viewed by the Hospital administration and physicians as essential, and could be defined objectively rather than in subjective or affective terms (Volland and German, 1979).

We were able to objectively define services as those required both to meet the needs of the Institution and at the same time the needs of patients. This was reinforced by our ability to communicate and demonstrate the positive outcomes of social work services to the directors and staff of the Functional Units. As a result, social work staff was increased to meet the identified needs of patients who needed help in making the transition from inpatient care to the community.

In the decentralized management system, social work service providers have the opportunity to market services to Functional Units. This means that the social work managers and staff are required to articulate the value of their services to the medical care programs provided for patients in each Functional Unit, i.e., Medicine, Pediatrics, etc. The ability to communicate these values is critical to the success of this process.

A second critical component of a successful marketing process is the ability to define social work services in such a way as to demonstrate that service delivery will ensure positive patient outcomes for the Functional Units. The Social Work Director is responsible for defining, designing, and implementing this marketing communication effectively.

This program required the use of knowledge deriving from many areas of social work training: social systems, group process, communications and human behavior theories. Particularly important is understanding the organizational structures of health care delivery systems, of health policy, and of legislative and regulatory measures, and financing of health care as these affect client utilization patterns. One particularly crucial skill is ensuring successful accountability measures within the system.

Understanding the organization of the Hospital is critical. A manager who is successful within an organization must accept the organization's direction and structure. An effective manager believes in the goals of the organization and demonstrates a commitment to these goals without any special interests predominating in this commitment. A manager of a professional department must protect the integrity of the specific discipline but not at the expense of a commitment to the overall goal of the organization.

Some professionals fall into a common pitfall when they place priority on the profession itself, rather than on what the profession can contribute to the organization's goals and success. When I first came to the Hospital, the President's view of social work was negative from his past experience; he saw social workers as concerned primarily about professionalism and only secondarily in supporting patient care needs through good social work practice. It is a crucial issue for the social work leader managing a professional service in a host setting. Unless the social work leader accepts the organizational direction and structure, the social work program may not be able to secure its proper role and place in the delivery of health care services.

A final important element for success is the social work director's ongoing and keen interest in health care, and how the health care system is changing. This interest in "the environment" allows one to anticipate change and begin to develop ways to ensure for social work's effective participation in this changing health care environment. Thus, it is not fortuitous that a program for social work administrators in health care, developed by the Society for Hospital Social Work Directors of the American Hospital Association, begins with the focus on helping the manager "read the environment." This is, in fact, the ability to utilize basic social work assessment skills learned in social work education and practice that must be applied generically to the health care field. The successful social work leader/manager utilizes these skills constantly in day-to-day work, and especially so during these times when health care delivery systems are changing rapidly.

Which of these elements did the Hospital leadership note in me as a basis for recognition, education, and promotion? The Hospital believes that good managers are leaders. The President recognizes and supports those managers who believe in the organization's goals, and who take the initiative to link their contributions to those goals with particular emphasis on demonstrating economic value. This ability to translate services into objective statements of outcome was instrumental in obtaining ongoing support of the social work service program (Volland, 1976). These services need to engender the respect of the medical and nursing professions as well as other care components of the Hospital.

Finally, opportunities for enhanced responsibilities within the organization need to be, and were available. Timing is a critical issue. At the time of my expressed interest in expanding my responsibilities, the Hospital was beginning to change its focus and direction. It was also interested in developing successful female managers. In summary, I was in the right place at the right time, and had demonstrated skills respected by Hospital management.

THE TRANSITION

Within five years of becoming the Director of the Social Work Department, I had developed and demonstrated interest in the broader health care system, including the efficient utilization of health care facilities and the improved delivery of services to patients in the community. I then initiated a discussion of future career alternatives with the President of the Hospital, who supported career advancement and recommended as a first step that I obtain an additional generic degree. I considered several alternatives before I decided to secure a Masters Degree in Business Administration. Supported and financed by the Hospital, I returned to school full-time while continuing my responsibilities as Director of the Department of Social Work. This arrangement continued for two full years. I was able to manage a full-time job and full-time student load primarily because the educational program occurred on weekends. Therefore, I worked full-time five days a week, and studied or attended school weekends and evenings. Business as usual occurred at the Department in the Hospital.

As this educational experience concluded, the Hospital was planning the organizational changes noted earlier. Hospital management positioned itself to provide more efficient patient care; to concentrate on strategies to control and expand the Hospital's patient care market; and to improve communication between Central Administration and the Functional Units. The process of reorganization valued and planned for the development of individuals with clinical and administrative talents for key management/leadership roles.

In this atmosphere of transition, my skills and desire for a career change were timely and congruent with the needs of the organization. Achieving the position of Director of the Department of Social Work of a major teaching hospital at an early age allowed me to think of further career alternatives; I did not believe that limiting my career development to the social work field in the future would be consistent with my expanded interest in broader health care issues. Therefore, the key for my continued career development was to plan for expanded and diversified areas of responsibility. I had had a consistent interest in broader health care issues, and was motivated to take on additional responsibilities. These intensified my desire for a position of greater influence on the systems of health care delivery. My basic social work commitment to provide quality services to patients and families, plus my demonstrated skills in developing and evaluating service delivery objectively, were considered important contributions I could make to the envisioned changes in management structure and style. Securing a Masters Degree in Business Administration with its associated financial skills and tools was considered by hospital leaders to be another useful preparation for the changes that were occurring in health care systems.

Other personal motivating factors included a continued desire to learn, to develop my management/leadership talents, and improve in areas of professional interactions. Achieving status and greater influence within the organization were strong motivating factors as were the economic gains associated with the promotion. Finally, I wanted to take advantage of having succeeded as a social work leader early in life. I saw that unless I gave serious consideration to a career change, future opportunities would be less likely to develop, and my motivation likely to decrease. The Hospital was committed to creating opportunities for talented women; this promotion to the senior management level would afford new challenges in fulfilling my professional career goals.

In summary, my own interests and motivations were known to the Hospital management. They supported the development of my career through education, and a reorganization occurred which could utilize the combination of skills and leadership I had developed. Since that time, my responsibilities have increased as I have demonstrated effectiveness in my new areas of responsibility. It remains a challenging opportunity.

There are advantages and disadvantages associated with a career change in the same institution. The social work staff initially expressed pride and a certain expectation that their interests were being protected. There was also an undercurrent that the change represented a ''sell out'' of social work values to personal ambition for increasing success. Former peers had other mixed responses to the change. It was difficult for them to accept my expanded role and increased authority. But it also gave them an opportunity to have increasing interaction with senior management. As Director of the Department of Social Work, it was clear that I needed to improve interpersonal skills especially with subordinates. This was a paramount concern in the transition. It became a major focus in developing relationships with directors of departments whose functions were not my areas of expertise. These managers also had a vested interest in developing a positive working relationship with me.

I did not retain the position of Director of the Department of Social Work. The President of the Hospital deferred to my recommendation to keep the positions and their associated responsibilities separate. I did not retain the Directorship because of a belief that to do so would diminish the value associated with the social work function in an increasingly changing hospital environment. The Department of Social Work needed a strong leader who could devote his/her efforts solely to insuring continued viability. To keep the title, in my opinion, would have given me personally more security at the Hospital; this security would, however, have been at the expense of the Department's continued development.

It would be impossible to talk about this transition and its changes without discussing the issue of women in senior management. This promotion had the potential to activate two biases: (1) about my being a social worker, and (2) being a woman. I concentrated my efforts on learning about the culture at this new level of management, and finding my place in a new role. I also concentrated in doing an effective job, and in good communication with peers and colleagues. These eventually resulted in my achieving a high level of personal comfort, and by others' acceptance of me in this new role.

APPLICATION OF SOCIAL WORK KNOWLEDGE, SKILLS, EDUCATION TO HOSPITAL MANAGEMENT

It is difficult to specify what social work knowledge, skills, and values have been most helpful in carrying out current responsibilities. Understanding human behavior and communicating effectively are critical skills. It is essential that one have respect for the integrity of other human beings whether they are patients or individuals with whom a manager must work in order to ensure effective service delivery. To complete important tasks associated with the management role, one needs to be aware of "where people are"—a clear tenet of the social work profession.

There are several significant knowledge areas described by Berkman (1978) that remain key to success in senior management positions. Basic is the ability to understand the health care delivery system and its financial aspects as well as health policy regulation in an ever changing environment. In order to demonstrate the impact of all services on the economic goals of the Hospital it is essential to use accountability structures effectively. Knowledge of legal and ethical issues as they are associated with the delivery of health care services is critical to patient care and hospital viability. As health care becomes more business oriented, management decision-making must take into account, much more than it did in the past, the meaning of illness to patients and families and its bio-psycho-social impact on their lives and functioning. Articulated as critical to social work practice in health care (Berkman, 1978) they are integral components of the processes of successful management decision making.

This knowledge and associated skills are now critical to the understanding and redefinition of "products" associated with effective health care delivery. For example, the way in which people react to dependency is a very important element in health care delivery, and becomes critical to ensuring patient satisfaction. Social workers have long known that people do well if they are able to return to familiar surroundings as early as possible. This has now become an economic necessity in the health care system, thus affording an additional opportunity for the use of social work expertise in health policy decision making.

My transition has been successful in part because a number of my skills were transferrable. Skills I had developed as a social work director have been extremely useful in this new position. This includes knowledge of the organization and its goals, the ability to work effectively with other people, and a commitment to assist in the development of the skills of other managers and colleagues. Understanding the health care delivery system is critical to generic management. Two personal qualities have proven to be especially useful. One is a constant motivation to learn new things, and the other is a willingness to acknowledge ignorance in order to learn.

From the outset, I focused my work with each new department or project for which I was responsible by working with staff to define its major contribution to the organization and its mission. This served to enhance the visibility of those departments and their projects to central administration, and to encourage diverse groups to work together more effectively, one of the goals of the reorganization. An additional benefit was the increased commitment of individuals in each of these departments from which ensued a greater recognition of their value to the organization. The ability to communicate effectively and interact with others thus becomes more crucial as one's responsibilities increase. This includes the ability to always make a point effectively whether orally or in writing (Heyssel, 1985). There were also new skills I needed to learn in this transition. Foremost are applying the tools learned in the program for a Masters Degree in Business Administration. Although I had been interested in financial and quantitative issues associated with successful business, my skills in this area were not developed prior to a return to school for this purpose. This educational experience was critical.

A vital new skill was learning to manage managers. A critical difference exists between managing supervisors in one's department, and managing managers who run their own departments. In the latter relationship, one is dealing with people who are used to making decisions in the areas they manage. To be effective, one has to learn how the managers manage, to become assured about their effectiveness, and to find ways to support their continued development while working with them to ensure commonality of goals. This requires a less directive approach than I had utilized previously as Director of the Department of Social Work.

It also required a change in assertive behavior. Assertiveness is a key positive behavior; however, when one directs a department such as Social Work, one is always committed to ensuring visibility and opportunities within the Institution so that the department can function professionally on behalf of patients. This requires significant assertiveness in an advocacy role. At the senior management level, with responsibilities and commitment associated with overall institutional development, one often needs to be less visible. The decision-making process must focus on people and bringing them together to ensure institutional success. One must become a facilitator who enables a variety of departments with some conflicting objectives to work effectively together to achieve the Institution's mission.

At this level, one learns quickly that one is not the only expert. One learns that more decisions are made through group process; in fact, a significant number of decisions do not always achieve clear closure. The management style of the President of the Hospital requires that people communicate effectively and develop abilities to work together. Boundaries are less defined and decisions often "happen" more than they are "made." This allows for continued growth and flexibility in an ever changing health care environment. It also requires a less directive or authoritative approach as well as a recognition that influence is subtle and exerted by those who are knowledgeable, competent in their jobs, and committed to effective communication. Managing ambiguity while insuring the motivation of others managers is a requisite skill.

This has been a very positive experience for me. Over the past three years there have been many opportunities to demonstrate my management and leadership skills in a variety of areas. Demonstrated effectiveness in meeting the expectations of an organization often results in acquiring new responsibilities. The organization continues to undergo change; this requires a commitment to keep up-to-date on the overall health care environment on a day-to-day basis. This is especially challenging.

As a woman in a senior management position, this experience has resulted in an increased sensitivity to assisting career oriented women to relate effectively with other women, and with the organization. Some men perceive that women are unable to work well together. This is not an accurate perception. However, it is critical for success-oriented professional women to demonstrate that they can work well with each other and with their male colleagues.

Each department in the Patient Services Division has been effective in defining and ensuring its contribution to the overall mission of the Hospital. Each department director is a capable manager of people, clear about the department's contribution to the Hospital, and flexible in meeting new challenges. As with any achievement, one must be prepared for the competition that naturally occurs. This is always a challenge. Finally, as a manager and leader, a most critical, ongoing responsibility is one's own continuing development, the ability to look critically at one's contribution and to identifying ways in which one can become more effective (Zaleznik, 1963).

CONCLUSIONS

I believe that there are opportunities present in the health care delivery system for those social work managers who seek to expand their careers. While much knowledge and many skills are transferrable from social education and practice, these alone will not be enough to ensure a successful transition. Especially critical is acquiring knowledge and skills to prepare one for financial and quantitated decision making, and for a business approach to health care delivery. This will have the added value of changing others' possibly stereotyped perceptions of social work. Above all, a successful transition will be likely if one focuses on managing one's responsibilities effectively in organizations that are changing daily to meet the challenges of staying in business in the health care industry today.

REFERENCES

Berkman, Barbara. *Knowledge Base and Program Needs for Effective Social Work Practice in Health: A review of the Literature, 1978*. Commissioned by The Society for Hospital Social Work Directors of The American Hospital Association.
Drucker, Peter F. *Management: Tasks Responsibilities—Practices 1974*. Harper & Row, Publishers. xiii.
Heyssel, R. M., Gaintner, J. R., Kues, I. W., Jones, A. A., and Lipstein, S. H. Decentralized Management in a Teaching Hospital. *New England Journal of Medicine*, 1984: 310,22: 1477–1480.
Heyssel, R. M. Personal Interview, 1985.
Volland, Patricia and German, Pearl S. Development of an Information System: A Means of Improving Social Work Practice in Health Care. *American Journal of Public Health*, 1979: 69,4: 335–339.
Volland, Patricia J. Social Information and Accountability Systems in a Hospital Setting. *Social Work in Health Care*, 1976: 1,3: 227–285.
Zaleznik, Abraham. *The Human Dilemmas of Leadership*. Harvard Business Review, 1963: 49–55.

CHAPTER XI

Social Work as a Preparation for Health Care Administration

Saul Zeichner, MSW, ACSW

CURRENT POSITION AND RESPONSIBILITIES

My current position is Vice President, Administration, Mt. Kemble Division of the Morristown Memorial Hospital. I was appointed to this position in March, 1985. Prior to this most recent promotion, I was Assistant Vice President, Community Services, a position held since 1978, having initially come to Morristown Memorial Hospital as Director, Social Service Department in July, 1975.

The Director of the Social Service Department reports to me administratively, along with the hospital and satellite Hemodialysis Unit, the Endoscopy Program, E.E.G., Chaplaincy Services, Geriatric Center, and all the hospital's mental health programs, which include Employee Assistance, Mediation, Psychiatric Emergency Services, Consultation and Education, and a number of other outpatient programs, including child abuse, and those affiliated with the Courts. In addition, I serve as the official liaison to the Departments of Internal Medicine and Psychiatry. In this capacity, I am available to solve problems as referred to me by the Chairman of Internal Medicine, but I am much more intensively involved with the Department of Psychiatry as the administration staff person providing program development and planning, grant writing and management, and program administration. I meet weekly with the Department of Psychiatry Chairman to review existing programs, identify and resolve problems, and plan and develop new programs. When I recently became the Administrator of our one hundred forty-eight (148) d step-down facility located three quarters of a mile from the acute care hospital, Endoscopy, E.E.G. and Chaplaincy Services were assigned to another Administrator.

One of my primary responsibilities is to represent the hospital in the community. The position was conceived as a formal liaison to the community to implement the hospital's increasing recognition that its walls needed to be extended. In this capacity, I represent the hospital on numerous social and health related agency boards throughout the County, as well as on the State and National level. For example, I serve on the following County or Agency boards: Drug and Alcohol Abuse, American Cancer Society, Retired Senior Volunteer Program, Inc., First Call for Help and Neighborhood House, to name just a few. At the State level, I serve on the Mental Health Committee of the New Jersey Hospital Association, and at the National level on the Section for Psychiatry and Mental Health of the American Hospital Association, from which I recently had to resign. I am also actively involved in program development, both by participating in long-term and strategic planning efforts of the hospital, as well as by developing new programs, writing grants, and seeking funding. The Center for Geriatric Care, funded by the Robert Wood Johnson Foundation Initiatives in Long-Term Care, is the most recent grant that I have helped to develop.

What has made my position most unusual is that I am held accountable for all of these assigned programs, but very few people report directly to me. Unlike product line management, in which the person responsible for the product line is also responsible for all its employees, hospital management tends to use a matrix system of management in which responsibilities are divided between the Administrative and Clinical functions (Galbreath, 1971). As a result, a staff person would report to their own Director for supervision of clinical functions, and to an administrative person for nonclinical functions, which is an inherent weakness in a Matrix system (Davis and Lawrence, 1978). In product line management, all of the people within the Unit would report to the Product Line Manager for all of their functioning and even those delegated areas such as professional supervision would still be the ultimate responsibility of the Product Line Manager. This is a very different form of administrative structure and has significant implications for the Health Care Administrator. In my instance, the Director of Social Work, E.E.G., the Geriatric Center and the Mediation Program were hired by and report directly to me, however, many of the other departments heads were neither hired by nor report to me. The Hemodialysis Department has a Medical Administrator, who is appointed by the Department of Internal Medicine, and reports to that Department. The Nursing Supervisor is responsible for the nursing staff and day to day operations of the unit and she reports directly to Nursing. I serve as the Administrator of the Unit, and am responsible to the Chief Executive Officer for its total functioning, with no direct control over any of the key personnel on the Unit. A similar situation tends to exist in Psychiatry where many of the staff report directly to a Psychiatrist in their Unit and the responsibility is divided between clinical and administrative functions. Since the definition of where administration stops and clinical begins tends to be very grey, it requires continuous negotiation to keep the programs moving. At the Mt. Kemble Division, where I am currently the Administrator and Chief Operating Officer, all the Department heads report to their immediate superior at the Madison Avenue Division. For example, the Director of Food Service at Mt. Kemble reports to the Director of Food Service at Madison Avenue, who reports to a different officer of the hospital. This lack of direct control has had a significant impact upon my management style and approach. In fact, my ability to negotiate results without direct power and control probably resulted in my original and subsequent promotions, and the realities of my work environment helped to further reinforce the skills.

THE TRANSITION

My first step into the world of administration was as the Director of the Social Service Department. Prior to that, I had interviewed for an administrative position on several occasions, but was not yet quite ready to leave the world of clinical practice. In fact, even as Director of the Social Service Department, I managed to keep an active caseload, not quite ready to make the full transition from clinician to administrator. It was only when several colleagues challenged me at a national conference that I resolved my ambivalence and made the first real move into administration. This transition remains a difficult one for clinicians and is probably the single most important issue to be resolved in the process of becoming an effective administrator.

Several key factors were responsible for my movement from social work to health administration. First, I accomplished my initial charge to change the Social Service Department without massive staff turnover and with a minimum of fuss. I came into a department staffed predominately by Bachelor Degree social work staff, and with all the Master Degree staff assigned to the mental health area. Focus was predominately on concrete services to the disadvantaged and poor. The majority of staff had been there a number of years, as had the previous Director. A counseling orientation was not strong within the department, and there was considerable fragmentation between the "medical social workers" and the "psychiatric social workers." The department was perceived within the institution as the people who dealt with money, determining how much a medically indigent person would pay, processing clinic cards, distributing clothing and other concrete items. The Departmental organization had not been changed for many years, and everyone was very comfortable proceeding with business as usual.

Recognizing where the staff were, I moved in slowly, focused on getting to know each of the staff, learning their strengths, and building upon them. I took the approach of involving staff in any changes within the structure. Being the newest person to a health care setting, I relied greatly upon their expertise and recognized that they had significant expertise to share. As the department progressed, new programs began to be developed, both through grants and through the hospital's initial willingness to make new staff available, so that the department began to move and grow and the staff felt a part of this process. Existing staff were assured they would not be replaced with Master's Degree people and that based on their experience and background they had much to contribute. At the same time, they were encouraged to go to seminars and develop and strengthen skills.

This does not mean that there was not a considerable stress in the process. Change is difficult for all of us and the staff experienced the change with difficulty, but there was sufficient and positive movement to help them deal with their feelings about change.

Second, since I had come from a mental health setting, I became the only non-physician administrator knowledgeable about mental health and psychiatric services and able to "speak the language." Up until that point, there had never been anyone in the hospital administration sufficiently knowledgeable to question requests for additional staff or to examine how clinical services were delivered. This immediately increased my value to the institution.

Third, within two years after my arrival at the hospital, I began to develop new programs and find additional funding. The Psychiatric Emergency Program was started when the psychiatrist in charge of the department did not get as much funding as she had sought and turned to me to develop an alternative program within the existing financial constraints. This was implemented successfully within the Social Service Department and has been operating ever since. I gained "points" by helping the Chairperson of Psychiatry out of a tough spot and by increasing admissions to the unit.

Fourth, I also began to serve a key role for the hospital President as I became better known in the community and could bring feed-back regarding community perceptions of the hospital. This community feed-back loop resulted in my periodically being placed in the position of advising the Chief Executive Officer not to proceed with a particular project despite his wish to do so, (something one does with caution). This gained his respect, expecially when time proved the decision to be accurate.

Fifth, was the ability to manage data in a coherent and concise manner and to support my position with numbers. This helped develop strong positive relationships with the fiscal personnel to the point that they developed confidence in my statistical justifications. Data was used to support requests for additional staff to increase the Social Service Department with some success, at least initially.

Finally, while accomplishments occurred within the institution, the President and members of the Board of Trustees also received positive feed-back from the community. All this helped me accrue an achieved status within the organization and to develop powerful allies from whom I could borrow power when needed (Linton, 1936). My achieved status which in itself contained little or no power, began to have power ascribed to the position as others recognized that I was "well connected." The ability to take an administrative position with little power in which almost no one reported directly to me and develop a source of power to accomplish the position objectives is critical to health care management. This point is well made by Wax (1968). As a result, when the hospital was planning an administrative reorganization, I received my first promotion in 1978, and I hired a new Director of Social Services.

I decided to accept this new position for several reasons. It provided the opportunity to participate more directly in health care policy and program development. This broader arena held more challenge and excitement than the day to day administration of the Social Work Department. The potential existed for me to have a broader impact on service delivery. Needless to say, it also paid a lot better, an important concern when sending children through college. The position also placed me closer to the decision making power within the institution with the perception that more could get done more quickly (not always necessarily so). Being closer to the top also makes one more vulnerable and stressed. There were also political factors which pushed my decision. If I failed to take the position, someone else would, to whom I would then report, and the person might not be someone with whom I could work well. Finally, there is often little choice in the decision to accept a promotion, since I, for one, could not really remain in the same institution and remain status quo. A final issue in moving into administration is preparedness. What did I know about health administration beyond one course in graduate school? Attempts to imagine my first day of work after this promotion came up blank. However, I quickly learned that in many ways my social work education and experience would prove helpful in the transition.

THE APPLICABILITY OF SOCIAL WORK KNOWLEDGE AND SKILLS TO MANAGEMENT IN HEALTH CARE

Since my graduate social work training was in the direct service track with heavy emphasis on both case work and group work, I had very little exposure to administration, community organization or social policy. I took the mandated administration course, but at the time, both because of my own orientation and also because of the way its content was presented, I did not get very much out of that course. Rather, I found that the generic social work knowledge and skills I acquired in graduate school and on the job were particularly helpful. Certain areas of knowledge and skill acquisition proved especially so when applied in a manner consistent with the objectives and functions of the new position. Those areas required in an administrative position include: (1) assessment of the people and system, (2) systems negotiation, (3) relationship building, (4) process/results orientation, (5) group skills, (6) community organization, (7) data management, (8) communication, (9) financial management, (10) power brokering, (11) interdisciplinary cooperation and, (12) time management and decision making. This list of skills and knowledge generally constitutes the content of most textbooks on administration. Some parts of the knowledge and skills base are currently conveyed in social work graduate education; some that are not I think ought to be a part of the curriculum. The next section addresses these knowledges and skills that are a part of existing social work curricula in graduate schools.

Assessment Skills

Textbooks in social work practice stress the need to develop assessment skills. Although Hollis (1964), Perlman (1957), and Hamilton (1951) represent different points of view, all three discuss the need for assessment-diagnosis as part of treatment. While in administrative work there is no one identified client being "treated," it is still essential to accurately assess people and situations in the hospital in order to select the most effective interventions. For example, it is extremely important to know how and when to bring an issue to the administrator. It is important to understand those areas that have priority and interest the administrator and those which turn him/her off. In bringing ideas to your administrator for consideration, one must build on the area of his/her interest, especially when you are seeking money to start a program. If you know that the administrator will not, or is less likely to, respond to emotional appeals about needy clients, then the program must be presented in a way which is more likely to get the desired response. Such an assessment is necessary to determine how to work successfully with a wide range of individuals: administrators, physicians, trustees, community agencies and committees. Developing sensitivity to where people are, to how to work most effectively with them, and when and how to intervene, become especially critical in a setting where you start with little power and control. Such an approach is consistent with social work training in assessment and the principle of starting where the client is.

Systems Negotiation

This is probably one of the most critical areas for administrative practice. Negotiation, the ability to work around, through and within systems, and to have the broadest view of systems and their interrelationships, is critical in moving from a social work management position to a hospital administrative position. Recognition of how systems fit together, their points of stress and their points of interaction, is required in order to know how to respond and intervene in them. This is especially important in health care administration where the administrator is held totally accountable for what happens in his/her departments, but frequently does not have direct control over anyone in those departments. Everything that is accomplished has to be through negotiation and developing relationships with individuals. This is accomplished by (1) helping them see that the administrator can do something for them to make their life easier, (2) facilitating the accomplishment of mutual goals, (3) enhancing their performance without loss of control or status, and (4) helping them to get their job done. In this sense, the administrator serves as a classic social work enabler and facilitator.

Relationship Building

Social workers are uniquely trained in developing and sustaining interpersonal relationships. The ability to be empathetic, to listen attentively, to sort out alternatives and to provide support, are primary basic skills developed during social work education, training and experience. They are skills that probably are most responsible for the movement of the social work administrator into health care management positions.

Process/Results Orientation

Social work literature is replete with emphasis on the concept of process. Pincus and Minahan (1973) discuss social work process in detail. The word "process" is used by field instructors as students do "process" recordings. Sometimes one feels we use the term ad nauseam. Yet, it is this very concept of orientation to process that makes social workers valuable in health care settings today. We, along with the human resources and personnel staff, tend to be the only hospital departments with a process orientation. Hospital administrators are trained predominately in a results orientation that is short on process. If you ask an administrator a question about what to do, he will generally tell you; if you ask a social worker the same question, you will be asked your thoughts about it and then be assisted in "processing" the issue. On the task-relationship continuum of Hersey and Blanchard (1976), administrators tend to have a high task-low relationship orientation while social workers tend to have a high relationship-low task orientation.

At the same time, this strength can also be an inherent weakness. There is often an obsessive focus on process, a kind of process for its own sake. In the rapid pace of health care settings there is no place for such a non-functional focus. Social workers' low task-high relationship orientation often creates tension between the Social Work Department and hospital administration. This is especially true in today's health care environment which requires "timely discharge planning" and an action results orientation in general. This has obliged Social Work Departments to develop a high task-high relationship orientation to achieve results without losing process. This is not something for which social workers are trained and this shift in orientation is stressful to social work staff as they try to retain the basic process and values system while getting things accomplished within pressured time strictures. However, our process orientation makes the social work profession unique in health care and it positions the director and the department in a strategic institutional role. Movement to a high task-high relationship orientation is central to good discharge planning and can strengthen the effectiveness of these critical activities of the Social Work Department. This movement is also particularly important if one wishes to make the transition from social work director to health care administrator.

Group Skills

Problem solving in health care increasingly occurs in small groups. With its increasing specialization, health care is an excellent example of the large knowledge organization described by Drucker (1966). A knowledge organization is one which is composed of workers who use their information, their thinking ability, their ability to synthesize and conceptualize in the performance of work, rather than physical or manual skills. In the health care setting, Drucker compares the hospital of yesterday with its few knowledge workers, a few nurses and the physician, supported by housekeeping, cooking, maids, aides, etc., to today's hospital with its proliferation of the health service professional; x-ray and lab technicians, dieticians, physical therapists, occupational therapists, and other therapists, social workers, etc. (Drucker, 1966). All knowledge workers are required to provide patient care, develop policy, or create new programs. Many of these activities take place in groups and to be effective groups need to have skillful group leaders and productive participants. John Wax (1968, 1983) has identified the key role an effective group member or leader can play in the decision making process. Training in group work has been particularly helpful to me in leading effective groups. Group skills help to keep the group focused while enabling participants to be involved in the process without feeling controlled or manipulated. Each person feels a sense of participation with the leader providing the traditional group functions of clarification, focusing, etc. Being a group participant or leader has frequently provided me the opportunity to serve as a decision making agent. That my group skills have been recognized has been evident through my frequent election to the Chair of community boards on which I serve. Leading productive groups results in members' retaining their motivation to participate in future groups (Larson, 1980). As a means to consensus building and decision making, group skills have proven to be important and valuable in my work, both in and outside of the hospital.

Community Organization Skills

Involvement in the community and work with other agencies have enabled me to identify health needs and to motivate other agencies to try to meet them, either alone, in combination with each other and/or in combination with the hospital. As I serve on many community boards, I am able to put together a broad range of information about how agencies interface with the hospital and to strengthen service delivery. For example, during a recent site visit, the Center for Geriatric Care was highlighted as an excellent community organization effort. The director of the program, also a trained social worker, worked with all of the many community agencies involved in service delivery to the elderly and helped them agree on common definitions, processes and procedures for case management services. Using community organization to develop networks among service providers is an area closely identified with social work practice.

Data Management

In the past, social workers were often exposed to research in a theoretical way which seemed to them unrelated to practice. My own research interest and graduate course work proved useful in that I acquired data management skills. The ability to organize data coherently and cogently in order to facilitate communication and to support a program concept or policy is critical in administrative work. Since administrators are swamped with paper, the ability to condense information to convey a message concisely is an important one. This is not an area in which social workers excel as they often tend to be wordy, general and somewhat unfocussed.

Communication skills have been helpful to me in making the transition to an administrative position, so I think they belong in graduate school curricula.

OTHER NEEDED SKILLS

This section addresses several other areas which I believe need to become an integral part of social work education.

Financial Management

The ability to manage numbers and to understand basic financial concepts is critical to strengthening communication skills and should be included in graduate social work education. One does not have to be an accountant or have a masters degree in business administration to be able to add and subtract, to understand benefit packages, to understand and even write a basic profit and loss statement, (or at least know what it is). In today's health care environment, with its competition and regulations, movement into administration is impossible without a basic understanding of budgets and this understanding is critical for the social work director. The need to cost out new programs, to communicate with financial staff in their language and to develop the Social Work Department into a revenue producing cost center has received much attention in social work literature (Rosenberg, 1980). In the present climate of cost reductions and prospective pricing, no new program can be advanced without at least an initial needs assessment and financial feasibility study, so that these skills must be taught and learned.

Power

John Wax (1968) has written about social work power and power in general. While I did not have assigned power, that is, the power to hire, evaluate and dismiss individuals who reported to me directly, I did learn how to develop power. Power is developed in several ways: (a) through doing favors and helping others, resulting in debts that can be called in when needed; (b) through the strength of personal relationships with many of the other departments within the hospital, such as maintenance, food service, housekeeping, security, etc., which are extremely critical to getting things done; and (c) through developing strong relationships with the Medical Director and the President of the hospital as back up when nothing else worked and I was pushed into a corner. They were available when I had a problem with a particular person and would ''lend'' me the use of their power when I had none of my own. This ''lending'' of power could occur in several different ways. This would occur by my discussing an issue with the Medical Director and/or President for "direction" as reinforcement to change the direction being taken by another person, who was unresponsive to my efforts to redirect them and discussions were unsuccessful. They would make the decision that what was being proposed was not acceptable and I would convey their feelings to the physician and tell him the decision that had been made. This has to be done with care but since these issues are routinely discussed in meetings, it is accepted as general proceedure. Another way would be to talk with the Medical Director and have him talk directly with the physician, or to call a meeting of a number of people including the Medical Director. On still another occasion, I was responsible for helping to save a hospital physician's salaried position; with this kind of action, one becomes perceived as having much more power and authority than one actually has. As a result, many of the physicians now recognize that I have power and therefore deal with me differently in the sense that since negotiation only occurs between equals, being perceived as having equal power changes the relationship and allows for negotiation of issues. However, it is important to use power appropriately, positively, and judiciously for success. A fourth way power is achieved is through developing a reputation for getting things done. Completion of projects in a way that helps others without self-aggrandizement results in strengthening one's position within the organization.

Interdisciplinary Cooperation

This is an area in which I have developed skills only recently. Because my original charge was to develop a strong central social work department in the first several years at the hospital, I did not interact as effectively as I might have with some of the other disciplines. This created some strained relationships, especially within the Nursing Department. However, over the last several years, I have begun to improve my interdisciplinary skills. Movement out of the social work directorship, and the broader perspective my new position required, helped me develop a more collaborative approach, especially as I became more secure in my new position. Reading Toffler (1980) and Drucker (1966) contributed to my better understanding of the issues in interdisciplinary cooperation. The concept of the wave theory clash and an understanding of the pre-learned behaviors which are antithetical to interdisciplinary cooperation have been particularly helpful. The fact that social work is only one of many disciplines in health care settings makes it critical that we learn more about the barriers to and skills needed for interdisciplinary cooperation. This critical skill is not taught specifically in the classroom or the field in many graduate schools, yet is essential for social work practice in health care where effective interdisciplinary collaboration is basic to service delivery.

Time Management and Decision Making

With the ever increasing work load expected of health care administrators and social work staff, effective use of time is critical. A successful manager needs to be both efficient and effective in getting the work done. Budget freezes and cutbacks require more work from the same staff and this requires a thoughtful examination of one's style of work and of how time is utilized and priorities established. An effective administrator is able to make decisions after accumulating and assessing all available information and then moves on to the next task. Rapid but informed decision making is often foreign to social work practice with its intensive focus on introspection, examination and selection of appropriate therapeutic interventions.

Communication skills are also important in effective time management. The ability to write and/or efficiently dictate brief but meaningful chart notes are essential skills for efficient and effective time management. It is time for graduate schools of social work to abolish long, hand written documents and to require a basic level of dictation skills. To insure that a document will be read, one must learn to present the content in a way that catches readers' attention and makes them want to read it. The development of skills in written and verbal communication is critical in both practice and management.

Readings

In addition to knowledge gained from formal education, certain readings have been particularly helpful to me in the transition from social work to health care administrator. Such readings in administration as Drucker (1966), Levy & Loomba (1973), Geneen (1984) and Blanchard & Johnson (1981), have been most helpful, as have such readings in health care administration as White (1981). In addition, two management seminars provided at the hospital broadened my knowledge base. Readings in the area of marketing have also helped broaden my orientation (Cooper, 1979) and (Kotler, 1975).

Political Experience

Another useful experience was my having been active in politics and having held public office as mayor of my municipality, where I was responsible for the overall management of the municipality including developing the annual and long-range budgets. I think that this experience sharpened my budget skills and developed my comfort with numbers, statistics and finance. Most recently, I have begun to increase my knowledge of computers, a needed technology in all areas of administration.

ENVOI

There were, however, some problems in this move. For example, it took a long time before I stopped being perceived by others in administration as a "closet social worker" and they began to see me as a hospital administrator. Some department heads often tended to see my being a social worker resulting in my favoring social work positions, rather than an administrator trying to perform an overall function for the hospital and hiring the best person for any particular position. Paradoxically, some of my own colleagues seemed unwilling to consider me any longer as a social worker, but thought I had "sold out to the other side." When I have presented at social work conferences some social workers in the audience have been quick to take the position that my movement into health care management was not a "promotion." I think suspicion and distrust of administrators often affects my relationship with my social work colleagues. In fact, some often refer to me as "having been a social worker," although I still think of myself as using my social work skills to function as a hospital administrator. I have identified for myself social work skills that have helped me to accomplish this move. I see myself as valuable to the profession in this position, in terms of the acknowledged recognition of how social work skills and education can contribute to health care settings, and as I represent social work in a position where I can potentially be more helpful to the profession. Certainly, a number of new programs that have been started at Mt. Kemble are programs with strong social work roots; many of them have resulted in the promotion of social workers within the hospital and the creation of new positions for social workers in the community.

There are times however, when it is an extremely lonely position. Part of this lies in the position itself, as administrators are placed so that a certain amount of loneliness is inevitable. Part of it lies in the sense of not really fitting in any one slot any longer. To some extent the feeling of really getting things accomplished and the added financial rewards compensate for that, but even there, though I am closer to the top, there is no magic in getting needed tasks accomplished; often they are not accomplished as quickly as fantasized. In a talk to field instructors, Garber (no date) once referred to the social worker as the "marginal person," one who neither identifies with the organization nor the client. The social worker who becomes a hospital administrator is perhaps a doubly marginal person. Finally, the whole question of whether my present position is transferable to another hospital or state remains in doubt. My suspicion is that despite my experience, it may not be transferable; not having an MBA or MHA may prove impedimental to my movement to another administrative position in the health care system. Reentry into a social work administrative position may also be difficult, both because of the loss in money and status, but also because I could be perceived as being "over qualified." This paradox may present a barrier to future job possibilities. It remains to be seen if those of us who have moved into hospital administrative positions without the graduate degrees can find similar positions in other institutions.

REFERENCES

Blanchard, Kenneth and Johnson, Spencer. *The One Minute Manager.* Berkley Books, 1981.

Cooper, Philip D. *Health Care Marketing,* Germantown, Maryland: Aspen Publications, 1979.

Davis, S. M. and Lawrence, P. R., "Problem of Matrix Organizations," *Harvard Business Review* (1978) 56(3): 131–142.

Drucker, Peter F. *The Effective Executive.* New York: Harper and Row, 1966.

Galbreath, J. R. "Matrix Organization Designs," *Business Horizons* (1971) 44(1): 29–40.

Garber, Ralph. "An Address to the Field Instructors," Rutgers University School of Social Work, New Brunswick, New Jersey, exact date unknown.

Geneen, Harold. *Managing,* Doubleday: New York, 1984.

Hamilton, Gordon. *Theory and Practice of Social Casework.* Columbia University Press, New York, 1951.

Hersey, P. and Blanchard, K. H. *Situational Leadership.* San Diego: Center for Leadership Studies, 1976.

Hollis, Florence. *Casework: A Psychosocial Therapy.* New York: Random House, Inc., 1964.

Kotler, Philip. *Marketing for Non-Profit Organizations.* Englewood Cliffs, New Jersey: Prentic Hall, Inc., 1975.

Larson, JoAnn. "Accelerating Group Development and Productivity: An Effective Leader Approach," *Social Work with Groups,* Vol. 3, No. 2, Summer, 1980, pp. 25–39.

Levy, Samuel and Loomba, N. Paul. *Health Care Administration: A Managerial Perspective.* Philadelphia: J. B. Lippincott Co., 1973.

Linton, Ralph. *The Study of Man.* New York: D. Appleton-Century Company, Inc., 1936.

Perlman, Helen Harris. *Social Casework: A Problem-Solving Process.* Chicago: University of Chicago Press, 1957.

Pincus, Allen and Minahan, Anne. *Social Work Practice: Model and Method.* Itasco, Illinois: FJEJ Peacock Publishers, Inc., 1973.

Rosenberg, Gary. "Concepts in the Financial Management of Social Work Departments," *Social Work in Health Care,* Vol. 5, No. 3, Spring, 1980, pp. 287–297.

Toffler, Alvin. *The Third Wave.* New York: William Morrow and Company, Inc., 1980.

Wax, John. "Clinical Contributions to Administrative Practice," *Social Work in Health Care,* Vol. 8, No. 3, Spring, 1983, pp. 129–139.

Wax, John. "Developing Social Work Power in a Medical Organization," *Social Work,* Vol. 13, No. 4, October, 1968, pp. 62–71.

White, Stephen L. *Managing Health and Human Services Programs, A Guide for Manager.* New York: The Free Press, 1981.

CHAPTER XII

Findings and Implications

In this chapter the editors identify patterns, themes, and issues that emerge from the contributors' collective experiences. We also examine their viewpoints and express our own about the role of social work education in preparation for management careers. Finally, areas for further study about the factors operative in social workers' mobility into management career paths are examined along with concluding observations and questions.

COMMONALITIES AND DIFFERENCES

As social work department heads, all the individuals whose experiences form the basis for the study understood and contributed to the overall mission of the institution in which they worked. They helped the organization fulfill its functions and goals in a visible way. This appears to have been central to their being tapped to make a continued and broader contribution.

Time and Place Opportunities

All first moved into hospital management positions in the same settings where they were social work managers. Such opportunities seem to have emerged and become available where (a) individuals were perceived as competent and capable social work managers; and (b) when there was congruence at a point in time between facets of the institution's needs and demonstrated human service skills.

All worked in hospital environments which in one way or another were fertile and hospitable for career progress. Most of these were reorganizing or expanding for greater efficiency, preparing for predictable and inevitable changes in the field of health care delivery. Sometimes, this occurred in conjunction with changing hospital missions and or with the development of new models of ambulatory, comprehensive care; sometimes, because of the specter of the impending financial crunch, and the need, imperative to survival, to plan ahead for more efficient organizations, new service programs and new links with the community to expand markets.

Many constituencies have articulated the need for increased attention to the human factors in health care service delivery. Social workers are particularly attuned to these factors. They are experienced not only in managing services but also in working collaboratively with physicians and other colleagues. They possess a unique combination of management and collaborative skills as well as sensitivity to patients, family and staff concerns, the sum of which put them in a good position to focus on the caring aspects of the overall hospital environment. Their movement into hospital management is natural and suitable.

All the contributors were recognized for some special competence: their productivity, management, planning and leadership skills were all above average, tested and visible, and seen as valuable to the institutions' missions.

As several note, they were ''in the right place at the right time.'' There was a ''person-environment'' fit in that their demonstrated capabilities were needed for their organizations' development.

Career Pathways

The contributors' approaches to securing executive positions in hospitals differed. Some note their desire to expand their spheres of influence and their arenas for action. Their pursuit of new positions was planned. Some did not seek out additional or changed responsibilities but took advantage of opportunities offered them as a result of their competence as social work managers. Some planned their moves subsequent to the first promotion.

Although some were more consciously planful than others, all freely acknowledged their ambition; they accepted and enjoyed challenges. Our impression is that no contributor to this book required assertiveness training.

Patterns of Their Continuing Relationships with Social Work Departments

In their transitions from social work to hospital manager, three patterns emerged.

In the first, the former social work director, now a hospital manager, retains responsibility for the operation of the department and actually holds dual positions reflected in their titles. This is true of four contributors, Bailis, Klingbeil, Rosenberg, and Simmons.

In the second model, the individual gives up the position of social work director, appoints a new director of social work who then has a reporting and accountability relationship to the ex-director, now hospital manager. Five started their executive careers in this pattern but moved to a third pattern. They relinquished both responsibility and accountability for social work as they moved into higher echelons or separate corporate entities. The social work department in these instances report to another administrator. This is the track followed by Flower, Goe, Light, Nielson and Zeichner.

Volland started with the first model, the dual role, and moved to the second. Now the director of social work reports to her.

Those in the first model saw advantages to the dual track of continued responsibility for the department, indeed, negotiated actively to retain it. They thought this a good way to retain their social work identity, both within the hospital and in the profession. They found this pattern either congruent with or integral to the potentially broader role social work can have in influencing hospital systems. They also believed it more advantageous for a social work department to work under the aegis of a hospital manager who is also a social worker than to report to a non-social work administrator. Lastly, some believed this pattern provides a safety net if the executive position is lost or threatened.

One complexity in this pattern is that the individual cannot give full time and attention to the care of the department, a factor which caused Volland to relinquish direct responsibility for it. Because of time pressures, the pattern is possible to maintain only if there is a strong person in the deputy director position and a strong departmental management team.

In model three the breadth and nature of the varied responsibilities seem to make both the direct or indirect connection functionally unfeasible.

We know from the work of Rino Patti (1983, 1979, 1979) that a move into administration implies in some sense, if only in the sense of risk, the possible loss or abandonment of values which have governed an individual's professional practice. The negative connotation seems to be intensified when the social work manager moves even further away from social work and becomes a hospital manager with no connection to the social work department.

Social Systems Perspective

All contributors brought an active, ingrained systems perspective to their work. Even those who emphasize the transferability of clinical skills used with individuals, families and groups to administrative problem solving use a social systems perspective. You can see the integration of this perspective in their thinking and their actions.

Each contributor explicated an almost reflexive response to the complex, interrelated components of the organizational matrix (Rosenberg and Weissman, 1981). All maintained a dual orientation and focus on needs of clients (patients and families) and the organization, were comfortable in responding to both systems simultaneously.

This dual perspective reflects a sophisticated form of advocacy which sees and assumes responsibility for meeting the needs of the multiple constituencies in both systems; for identifying where needs are congruent and mutually advantageous; for helping each use the other since each needs the other (Schwartz, 1961); for noting conflicts and differences in meeting the needs of both; for coalition building; and for helping both systems move to accommodation and equilibrium with each other.

Goe notes the need for a high level of understanding of social systems and environmental interaction, pinpointing the concept that if one views the entire hospital as a social agency, the missions of the social work department and the hospital are not dissimilar, although their priorities may be. It appears that understanding of these similarities and negotiating to find common ground is habitual within these executives.

This knowledge of social systems, with its varied views from multiple windows, is emphasized by all, whether it is specified as a vital ingredient for effecting change; in the use of organizational data; or with models promulgated on ecological systems, systems theory and theories of person-environment fit.

Applicability of Social Work Knowledge and Skills to Management Functions

Each contributor emphasizes the usefulness of social work skills in their performance as managers. All started in their careers as clinicians whose skills they report were applicable in their expanded management responsibilities and roles.

A list of useful values, knowledge and skills could provide an outline for a book on social work theory and practice (See Appendix I).

The common thread and key point seems to be the appropriate match of social work knowledge and skill to the situation. For example, in a meeting to review fiscal and budget issues, social work skills are not likely to provide much help. But in a meeting devoted to establishing program priorities for resource allocation, social work values can help. Social work skills are useful in management functions where assessment of people and systems figure significantly.

Finding the analogue of the study, diagnosis and treatment processes in organizational problem solving; or finding the program planning analogue in marketing; assessing both needs and wants; developing products or services, promoting them, evaluating them and refining them; this is the nature of the process of applying clinical skills to the macro level. It is seen by all as important.

Some contributors believe a solid base of social work knowledge and skill is all that is needed for success in management. Some emphasize the usefulness of social work skills in combination with other management skills. A third group thinks social work is essentially useful but not a requirement for management positions.

Five contributors noted problems posed by the use of some social work skills. Bailis thinks the passivity of good clinicians, with their "therapeutic neutrality," is not so valuable in management tasks. Adherence to the value of patience with process and of client self-determination often can impede and delay decision-making. A hospital manager needs a dual focus on process and results; Zeichner notes that social work is strong in the first, less suited for a results orientation. Nielson notes that the concept of self determination can sometimes impede the executive functions in management. Involving employees and staff in decision making is not always possible and may be an obstacle. Light identifies qualities that make for a good clinician, i.e., listening with the third ear, social perspective, working with conflict, etc., but sees them as disadvantages in the management of institutions that are "principally a workshop for medical practitioners."

Often the indirect, dynamic techniques useful to clinicians are not suited to the administrative need for a more direct, decisive management style where the manager has to take an unpopular decisive stance and give up "the luxury of a facilitating approach" says Goe.

Preparation for Management Role

It has been pointed out (Patti, 1979) that in the move from direct service to administration, practitioners frequently believe that their analytic and inventive skills will prove a sufficient armamentarium for management tasks. However, these managers often lack an organizational perspective: they need to learn about organizations and systems and to acquire other management skills. Social work directors who move to hospital manager positions clearly need to acquire a different, additional set of skills to deal with multiple departments and multiple functions.

The new content areas were:

1. *Financial Management*
   Financial analysis and planning, cost accounting, budgeting, reimbursement mechanisms, data processing and dealing with quantitative data.
2. *Monitoring, organizing and controlling functions*
   Establishment of accountability patterns; measuring productivity

and efficiency; understanding the differences between line and staff functions with ability to perform both.

3. *Strategic planning and marketing*
   Establishing short and long range goals; using 3–5 year time horizons; shifting from tactical to strategic planning.

4. *Time Management*
   Managing multiple demands on one's time. Establishing and adhering to priorities about the use of one's time.

5. *Decision Making*
   Influencing decision making processes; making decisions with or without others' input; knowing when and how to make rapid decisions.

6. *Negotiating*
   These include power brokering, use of management "language" instead of social work jargon; improving collaborative skills; helping subordinates in their development.

Although they agree on content, they differ on its significance: belief that this knowledge and skill base was not only requisite, but exceeded those of social work in importance; at the other end of the spectrum, belief that the application of social work skills in the new situation was the major help in their basic adaptation. However, all acknowledged the need to acquire additional knowledge.

The contributors used two routes to acquire this: (1) degree related formal education and (2) continuing education via courses, workshop and seminars. There was no consensus about the need for formal degree credentials. Volland completed an MBA with her institution's support. Nielson, Bailis and Klingbeil terminated their formal post graduate education just short of acquiring the degrees. Rosenberg had a doctoral degree in organizational development and the sociology of complex institutions at the time he became a director of social work. Others acquired no formal credentials in administration or finance but learned them on the job, and through courses and seminars. This was not a problem except in establishing credibility with some colleagues. Some found a mentor and/or gathered subordinates strong in formal administration and finance training. All became readers, stayed au courant with the literature on management, hospitals, finance, etc, and attended seminars and conferences. Some teach management.

Transition Management

Beckhard and Harris (1977), writing on organizational development, consider the management of transition states the most complicated of management tasks. They suggest that even though we know where we are and where we want to go, management of the journey calls for crucial skills.

This, of course, is not a new concept for social workers who are in touch with the many transitional issues which arise in the moves from clinician to supervisor to manager, and who have developed a body of literature on the dynamics and processes of the changes involved. In these ten narratives, we can identify other transitional hurdles many had to negotiate. These common issues can help others in their preparation for similar changes.

What were these transitional problems and how were they resolved? How did these individuals who moved into management echelons outside of social work deal with their conflicts about leaving what is known, whether it is comfortable or not, and moving into the unknown, no matter how desirable it seemed?

Dealing with the reactions of their social work staffs was common work. In varying degrees, they had ambivalent reactions reflecting fears of desertion and possibly competitiveness on the one hand, and, on the other, increased feelings of security (we'll be better protected), pride in a colleague's advancement and optimism that similar opportunities might exist for them. Often these reactions reflected reality concerns that those who retained responsibility for the direction of the social work department would give less or insufficient time to it. Such reactions are valid and need to be accepted as "normal," lived through and endured, as realities are separated from fantasies. The fact is that working relationships with professional colleagues will change as functions change.

More difficult to deal with are charges of abandoning the profession, of moving into "business." Social workers are often pejorative about colleagues who move outside of social work structures and agencies. Silberman (1984) notes that while lawyers are always lawyers, and physicians always doctors even if they are administrators, social workers often see colleagues who move into management as giving up their identity as social workers.

This issue of professional identity confronted this group as they moved from an unambiguous role to a broader one. For example, Bailis notes that while social work does not have a monopoly on caring, the social worker as manager has a particular conflict when the option and vote is either the patient's or the hospital's interest. This conflictual theme is expressed by the other contributors. Nielson sees the role of patient advocate a handicap to a hospital manager. Colleagues charged him with being "too emotional," a "typical social worker," not a "true administrator" as he negotiated for the rational deployment of resources. In any social work position, the advocacy role is unambiguous. Social workers are expected to provide balance to the institution's self interest and to emphasize the patient's interest.

A major theme is the struggle to reconcile social work values with the "bottom line" imperative. For example, a value conflict may arise around a marketing plan geared to attract a higher socio-economic group of consumers. The hospital's survival demands this, but there is an implication of less good for some clients. How does one balance the needs and rights of the client system (advocacy) and that of the organization? Light believes the rigors of financial constraints in health care settings will intensify this conflict for social workers perhaps to the point of untenability.

In successful transitions, it appears that a new professional "identity" is achieved over time: the contributors are administrators who are also social workers. New skills and old social work ones are blended successfully.

Along these lines, hospital staff other than social workers sometimes greeted the contributors' entry into management with ambivalence, sometimes with stereotypical accusations of being "bleeding hearts" and "do gooders," sometimes with accusations of favoring social work over other departments in allocating resources, sometimes with charges of lack of preparation and credentials in management and finance, part of the price of promotion in the same setting.

As our contributors struggled to carve out their identities in these new roles, they often felt lonely and alienated, with a sense of belonging to neither group. They needed to assume a new identity and role, a new profession. It is important to note that two of the ten contributors, Klingbeil and Simmons, moved into broader roles without experiencing this alienation.

Conflict and loss in giving up clinical work was common. This transitional issue is also characteristic of movement from clinician to director in social work programs but it seems to be more complex in the shift to broadened roles. Some often wished to return to clinical social work or to the social work department as their primary base.

The shifting from a process to a results orientation was problematic. The higher yield reward as social work clinician diminishes in the position of social work manager and lessens even more so as hospital manager. One needs to postpone rewards and look to long range success. One needs to exercise authority in new ways; to readjust one's leadership style; to make peace with the fact that involving employees in decision-making is not always possible. Most found they needed to adopt a more decisive management style; clarity as to when to make decisions on their own, when to involve others in them. They needed to learn the benefits and limitations of power, the difference, as Nielson says, between "getting things done right" (a seductive trap) and "getting the right things done."

They had to cope with gaps in their knowledge base and to be comfortable in acknowledging them as they gained the new base for themselves and worked with others who could provide the skills and expertise they lacked.

Significant in these transitions is the need to deal with the new and often unfamiliar authority entailed in management of disciplines other than one's own, and the handling of conflicts among different professional groups. A larger question is whether the broad range of professionals represented in a complex hospital system can be "managed" with any degree of consistency. Effective health care management frequently depends upon loose implementation structures which rely heavily on the performance of other people over whom the manager has little direct professional authority. How, for example, does a non-medical manager "manage" the Chief of Surgery and his department?

For some of the women contributors, gender posed an additional hurdle in career advancement. Stereotypes often prevail, such as the notion that women are more emotional, less business-like than their male colleagues. Some women social workers in management positions have more difficulty than their male colleagues in gaining acceptance by other managers because stereotypes of social workers are sometimes compounded with gender issues: it is hard for women to "break into" the "boys' club" (Kanter, 1977). Networking may be more difficult for them. The process of being accepted as managers in a field where men predominate both as administrator and physician poses a complicated transition for women. Salary equity is rare. To cope, attributes of both assertiveness and equanimity are required.

Subsequent Mobility

Five of the ten contributors, Light, Flower, Goe, Nielson and Bailis have moved from the institutions where they were first promoted to executive positions in other organizations. A question for the rest is whether the knowledge and skills acquired in taking up new responsibilities are transferrable to other institutions.

Most felt it would be untenable to "fall back" to the position of manager of social work. Thus, the question arises of whether formal additional credentials (MBA, MHA) would act as some measure of insurance for the continuation of a career in hospital management.

Light thinks those in hospital administration have short lives because, as he suggests, any administrator "who does not control the means of production (MDs who admit patients to the hospital) and who is powerless to establish price (reimbursement is set by others) is doomed to failure." He is not sanguine about opportunities for social workers to become institutional executives.

Summary of Personal Qualities and Motivation

Can we pinpoint what motivated these individuals to move beyond the management of social work services? Can we identify their personal qualities?

Some are stated, some implied: they are ambitious, have a capacity to take on risks of the unknown, of failure, of rejection. Clearly, they are hard workers, could not have achieved their positions working a 7–8 hour day. They had tenacity, could tolerate ambiguous identity and often ambivalent acceptance by others.

All are articulate and analytic. They possessed demonstrated leadership and management skills. They had conviction about what social work can and should contribute to an organization by applying knowledge of patient/family needs to humanizing the service delivery systems of a hospital.

Some sought expanded action options, wanted to stretch their capacities, liked and needed challenges. Some wanted to move ahead, earn more money, gain power, influence and authority, combine concern with individual needs to policy and program development for populations.

Others wanted to influence patient care directly and globally through access to resources. They wanted to be at decision-making levels and have some influence on decisions. Some wanted to see more rapid results. Some liked the variety of combined functions of administration, teaching and direct service.

They wanted the chance to use their skills in a larger arena and to demonstrate social work's usefulness to management tasks. Simmons believes social work function is broader than the provision of direct services and includes interventions to influence the institution's ambience. Rosenberg wanted to test whether he could remain a director of social work and carry a management position in a large hospital. Could he help create a therapeutic environment? Light thinks that "each of the moves in (his) natural progression towards positions of greater responsibility was rationalized on the basis that by the nature of (his) position in the organization, they could lead to greater humanization of the health care delivery system."

DATA SUMMARY

Generalized characteristics of the experiences of the ten contributors:

1. Each first moved into hospital management positions in the settings where they were first social work managers. This suggests that there may be an inherent set of management opportunities for social work directors in their own institutions.

2. Some planned their entry into broader management responsibilities and some took advantage of opportunities offered to them. Whatever the pathway, they had recognized, visible and tested special competencies as social work managers, planners and leaders. This suggests that competencies in social work management are transferable to other management functions.

3. As they took on broader functions, some retained responsibility for managing the social work department and some relinquished these ties. It is difficult to draw conclusions in this area. Both patterns are viable: they constitute a continuum, however an individual moves along it, and one can stop at any point. The exact factors that make for the differences cannot be pinpointed. Certainly, all participants are ''committed'' to social work, so that commitment per se cannot be the determining variable. Other organizational factors may be influential, such as the political and economic climate, transitional imperatives and marketing perceptions of legitimacy. Issues of power may also be operative. One can see continuing relationship with social work departments as enhancing power because social work provides direct access to knowledge of consumers' needs, just as one can view developing and expanding services to clients as accrual of power which can lead to promotion.

4. All used a social systems perspective in their work and maintained a dual focus on the needs of patients/families and of the organization, responding to both sets of systems simultaneously. This dual perspective appears to be a requirement for movement into hospital management, indeed for success in social work management. Social workers are among the few generalists in increasingly specialized professions. The usefulness of this generalist training comes through strongly.

5. A range of social work knowledge and skills used in clinical assessment and treatment were applied to the broader perspective of hospital and community systems. It appears that many of the skills which make for expert clinicians also contribute to managers' expertise, be they social work or hospital managers. They make for a dynamic way of processing and analyzing human interaction and concrete data for effective problem assessment; for developing plans and strategies; for teasing out options; for resolving conflicts; for managing people and operations; and for evaluating services and fiscal outcomes.

6. Conversely, some social work attributes (neutrality, process orientation) and values (self determination) have potential for posing problems in executive functions. The need to achieve a flexible balance of process and results orientation is a predictable transition task.

7. Movement into hospital management brought with it the need to acquire additional knowledge and skill for effective functioning in the new activities. Many of these are also needed for social work management. Some contributors obtained formal degree credentials, others used less formal routes for skill expansion.

8. Individuals who move from social work administration to hospital management can expect to encounter transitional problems, issues and conflicts. The nature of these hurdles can be anticipated, learned and taught. Issues that arise with some regularity are: colleagues' reactions; ambiguous professional identity; place of client advocacy; loss of rewards associated with the clinical role; balance of process and results orientation; uses of authority; and acceptance of women in a predominantly male domain.

9. All contributors displayed leadership and management capabilities as well as ambition, tenacity, and capacity for hard work. These personal qualities were buttressed by motivation for greater impact on the how health services are delivered, greater access to resources, a chance to use their skills in a larger arena and demonstrating social work's applicability and usefulness to the management of hospital systems.

10. The five that have moved in their career paths to executive positions in institutions other than where they were originally promoted suggests that it is feasible to maintain this career choice over time.

IMPLICATIONS: GRADUATE SOCIAL WORK EDUCATION AS PREPARATION FOR MANAGEMENT POSITIONS

Can we draw conclusions from the contributors' experiences about the need for curricula changes in graduate school of social work? Should additional content be added to prepare social workers for careers in management?

Some think that generic social work education combined with an integrated skills base prepare one for a host of opportunities and options; and that this generic base is especially useful in management positions, as their own careers demonstrate. They believe that no additions to current graduate school curricula are needed. They think technical knowledge of management can be added later, as needed in specific situations.

Others believe that social work curricula should be strengthened by greater emphasis on organizational theory and on the management of organizations. They think this content is needed to broaden the often limited perspective of clinicians. Specifically, a content base of how to work with power structures and of how to develop strategies for negotiation are seen as content relevant to organizational theory.

Between these two positions is the viewpoint that more basic management knowledge would be useful for all social workers at all levels. For example, knowledge of strategic planning can help position social work programs effectively and place social work expertise in the service of the organization; even though social work services are soft services, a management perspective can put a "hard" value on them.

The editors observe that graduate social workers interested in moving into administration, whether in or outside of social work, already have a choice of several post masters' sequences in social work administration or in post graduate business schools. Social work graduate education needs to remain generic in its concentration on micro and macro systems, methods and social policy content, the curriculum which makes social work education unique and clearly provides the particular constellation of skills in relation to system building which contributed to the initial success of the study participants.

However, as Patti (1983) points out, social workers are ill prepared for the transitional processes that normally occur in social work, that of moving from clinician to supervisor to manager. What needs to be strengthened in social work master's programs are areas of financial management, financial accountability and general management skills to provide a basic level of knowledge useful to all social workers, a base which could be supplemented by later education appropriately specific to job tasks.

AREAS FOR FURTHER STUDY

These findings are a beginning in our understanding of the phenomenon of social work managers' movement into positions of broader hospital management. But, as is characteristic of exploratory studies, they raise many questions for further study.

1. Why do health care organizations select social workers for management positions? How open is the field? It would be useful to learn directly from hospital executives why they have (or have not) selected social workers to join top management teams. What is *their* perception of social workers' management capabilities?
2. What is the total population of social workers who have moved into hospital management? A national survey of hospital managers could tell us how many are social workers.
3. What are the differences and similarities between hospital managers originally trained as social workers (MSW) and those trained in management (MBA, MHA)? A comparative study of the behaviors of managers in each group would address this question.
4. What organizational factors' or individual characteristics (or both)

are the crucial variables in the different patterns of continuing relationships which hospital managers who were first social work
managers have with their hospital social work departments? This
question can also be addressed by a comparative study of the two
groups, those who continue to manage hospital social work departments and those who do not.

5. What is the impact of economic pressures, leaner times and less
   altruistic approaches to decision making on the social worker who
   has become a hospital manager? What value conflicts arise? How
   are they resolved?

6. Will those who moved into hospital management in the last decade
   continue in this career in the next? This can be explored in a
   longitudinal study of our contributors and others at 5, 10 and 15
   year intervals.

THEIR FINDINGS AND OURS

1. Patti (1983) notes that the movement into social work administration continues to be one of the few options open to social work
   practitioners seeking increased status and salaries. We have found
   this motivation holds for many of the social workers in this study.

2. Patti (1979) also points out that social work clinicians who move to
   social work management believe that social work knowledge and
   skills are useful and needed in the management of social work
   organizations. This study confirms that they are certainly useful in
   hospital management. But other kinds of knowledge and skills in
   management are needed as well.

3. The question of whether social work education should include
   content in management skills is still being debated. Neugeboren
   (1986) deplores the fact that the ''social work education system
   persists in educating primarily for direct practice in spite of
   manpower needs for professional social workers trained in administration and supervision.'' Our study indicates that clinical skills
   are important to humanistic management and are not so certain that
   the classic social work curriculum should be changed. Nor do we
   agree with Saari (1975) who suggests that knowledge and skill in
   clinical practice may be antithetical or dysfunctional for social work
   administration and policy development. The findings of our study
   suggest that the social workers who are now hospital managers
   found clinical practice helpful in their new roles.

4. Patti and Austin (1977) note role discontinuity, identity confusion
   and concomitant stress in social work clinicians who become
   managers. What is interesting in our study is that our contributors

had less problems with these transitions, possibly because many of the developmental tasks Patti and Austin identify have already been mastered; and because their transition to new hospital management roles took place with negotiations of these transitional tasks already successfully completed. This is an impressionistic observation which would need to be confirmed by future empirical studies.

5. Each of the contributors agree with Patti (1983) that the person should be particularly aware that administration itself is a professional activity and requires at least the same level of expertise and dedication required of clinical practitioners. This recognition may be in part responsible for their success. It accounts for their immersion in additional training and for their ability to analyze their management behaviors (Levenson and Klurman, 1972).

6. Patti (1983) thinks that practitioners who become managers of social work programs frequently lack an organizational perspective. Our contributors all agree that a systems perspective is a sine qua non for hospital management.

7. It seems evident to us that the contributors to this study had already achieved some degree of mastery in their effective use of administrative authority. In their transitions from social work to hospital management, authority issues seemed to pose few problems for them. They transferred already learned skills in this area. This was true with both the authority derived from professional accountability and the authority which rested on collaborative accountability. The contributors' pattern was to first develop comfort and skill in the uses of their professional authority as social workers practicing in collaborative settings; and then to develop comparable ease in using their administrative authority as social work managers. The combination of both underpinned their ability to make valued contributions to their institutions. They understood, too, the limitations of their formal power and the potential power which can be derived by influencing, educative and planning strategies.

Finally, the setting and the individual, and their influence on each other, may be the crucial variables for social workers' movement into hospital management, a concept of social ecology quite familiar to social workers.

Gary Rosenberg, PhD
Sylvia S. Clarke, MSc

REFERENCES

Beckhard, Richard and Harris, Reuben T. *Organizational Transactions: Managing Complex Change.* Addison-Wesley Publishing Company, Reading, Mass., 1977.

Kanter, Rosabeth M. *Men, Women and the Organization.* New York: Basic Books, 1977.

Levinson, Daniel J. and Clurman, Gerald L. "The Clinician Executive," *Administration in Mental Health,* Winter, 1979, pp. 53–67.

Neugeboren, B. "Systems Barriers to Education in Social Work Administration," *Administration in Social Work,* Volume 10, No. 2, Summer, 1986, 1–14.

Patti, Rino J. "Social Welfare Administration," *Managing Social Programs in a Developmental Context.* Englewood Cliffs, N.J.: Prentice-Hall, 1983.

Patti, Rino J. et al. "From Direct Service to Administration: A Study of Social Workers Transitions from Clinical to Management Roles," *Administration in Social Work,* Vol. 3, No. 2, Summer, 1979, pp. 131–151.

Patti, Rino J. et al. "From Direct Service to Administration: A Study of Social Workers Transitions from Clinical to Management Roles, Part II, Recommendations," *Administration in Social Work,* Vol. 3, No. 3, Fall, 1979, pp. 165–275.

Patti, Rino J. and Austin, Michael J. "Socializing the Direct Service Practitioner in the Ways of Supervisory Mangement," *Administration in Social Work,* Vol. 1, No. 3, Fall, 1977, pp. 267–280.

Rosenberg, Gary and Weissman, Andrew. "Marketing Social Services in Health Care Facilities," *Health and Social Work,* Vol. 6, No. 3, August, 1981, pp. 13–20.

Saari, Rosemary C. "Effective Social Work Intervention in Administrative and Planning Roles: Implications for Education," in *Facing Challenge:* Plenary Papers, New York Council on Social Work Education, 1975, p. 43.

Schwartz, William. "The Social Worker in the Group," *Social Welfare Forum.* New York, Columbia University Press, 1961.

Silberman, Samuel J. "A View from the Sidelines," Council on Social Work Education, Thirtieth Annual Program Meeting, Second Plenary Session, March 12, 1984, Detroit, Michigan.

APPENDIX I:
SOCIAL WORK KNOWLEDGE AND SKILLS APPLICABLE
TO MANAGEMENT FUNCTIONS

Values

— Right of individuals to self determination;
— Principle of equal access.

Knowledge

— The dynamics of behavior of individuals, families and groups;
— The political nature of decision making;
— Understanding systems and organizational behavior;
— The dynamics of effecting change;
— Small group theory.

Skills

— empathy;
— interviewing and eliciting skills;
— skills in listening and clarification;
— understanding non-verbal communication, skill in responding to latent as well as manifest content, to stated and hidden agendas;
— starting where the individual, group or community is;
— skill in the study and assessment process;
— ability to establish good interpersonal relationship with a variety of people;
— ability to understand issues from different points of view;
— skill in understanding and facilitating small group processes;
— skills in advocacy;
— skills in negotiating systems;
— collaborative skills;
— diplomacy;
— comfort and skills in mediating differences, and dealing with conflict;
— skill in negotiating linkages for client and organizational needs;
— skill in program planning;
— skill in the uses of direct and indirect power; ability to negotiate results without power;
— capacity for self-awareness, self-analysis and introspection.